Revised Edition

Diet *in* Diseases

Sunita Pant Bansal

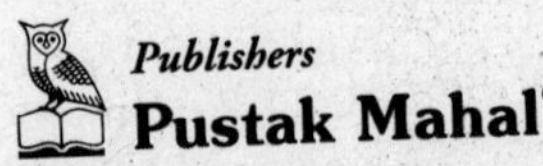

Administrative office and sale centre

J-3/16 , Daryaganj, New Delhi-110002
☎ 23276539, 23272783, 23272784 • *Fax:* 011-23260518
E-mail: info@pustakmahal.com • *Website:* www.pustakmahal.com

Branches
Bengaluru: ☎ 080-22234025 • *Telefax:* 080-22240209
E-mail: pustakmahalblr@gmail.com
Mumbai: ☎ 022-22010941, 022-22053387
E-mail: unicornbooksmumbai@gmail.com
Patna: ☎ 0612-3294193 • *Telefax:* 0612-2302719
E-mail: rapidexptn@gmail.com

ISBN 978-81-223-0814-3

Edition: 2017

Printed at : Sunny Offset, Delhi

Dedicated

to

Ma

Acknowledgement

As soon as my first book, *Healing Power of Foods*, came out in the market, I felt the need for discussing the role of foods or diet, in relation to any disease, getting stronger. It is very important to understand the disease, and how and where it affects the body, before any diet is prescribed for it. My first and foremost thanks to Ram Avtarji for understanding this and encouraging me to write on my favourite subject.

Thanks are due to Sujith, for typing the manuscript.

I am blessed to have a family that not only encourages me constantly, but also gets more excited than me on my achievements — thanks to Avdhesh, Shruti, Smriti, Sunil and Ritu!

Lastly, thanks to my mother, whose absolute, unconditional support and encouragement in everything I do is what gives me the confidence to aim for and achieve more and more in life.

Sunita Pant Bansal
NOIDA, U.P.

January 2003

Contents

Introduction

For many people, 'diet' is synonymous with weight reduction. People, mostly girls, are heard saying, "I am on a diet" or "I am dieting these days", which really means that they are on a weight-reducing diet. In fact, very few people realise the importance of diet. Diet actually includes everything that a person eats — be it more or less, good or bad. Diet means food, and it has a very important role in man's struggle against disease and debility.

It is well known that a 'balanced diet' is necessary to maintain good health; at the same time, one should also realise the importance of proper diet when the body is diseased. An appropriate diet would help the diseased body to move faster on the road to recovery. For every kind of disease or physiological disorder, the regular diet is modified to form a special therapeutic diet, which reduces the burden on the diseased organ and relieves the symptoms and other manifestations of the disease.

Therapeutic diets have an important role in modern medicine. Many patients do not get adequate advice and instructions, and as a result, they may fail to derive full benefit from the other forms of treatment. Doctors seldom prescribe full dietary instructions. For example, a patient with ulcers or typhoid would be prescribed a 'bland diet'. Since it is left to the patient to go into the details of the diet himself, he would just end up avoiding only spices. The diet therapy being incomplete, the symptoms would not be totally relieved, resulting in relapses.

In the same case, a dietician would explain to the patient in detail about the thermally, mechanically and chemically bland foods. Such a dietary instruction would help cure the ulcers or typhoid quickly and automatically relieve the symptoms.

Almost every disease is related to diet. Some diseases are caused by improper diets, and some require modifications in the diet as a part of their treatment.

Under-eating or under-nutrition leads to deficiencies of various nutrients, anaemia being the most common of such deficiency disorders. Loss of hair and skin problems are also related to the deficiency of certain vitamins in the diet. Obviously, to rectify these problems one has to rectify the diet.

Some people are under the wrong impression that health depends on the quantity of food eaten. Over-nutrition actually results in obesity. A little over 100 calories extra per day, that is, one banana or a fistful of peanuts or a plate of idli, would result in ½ kg gain in body weight over a period of 4-5 weeks. This would mean an increase of 5-6 kg in body weight in a year! Obesity brings with itself a number of other complications like heart disease, joint pains, respiratory problems, to name a few. In order to combat all these problems, a diet is required — a reducing diet in this case.

Physiological problems such as the fevers of typhoid and tuberculosis etc., liver and kidney disorders and other problems associated with our body systems, also require diet modifications. The modifications are made so that the impaired organs of the body are given rest, and so the medication is more effective.

Dietary changes are needed in periods of physiological stress like pregnancy and lactation (breastfeeding the baby). Dietary requirements also change as we grow up. They are different for babies, children, teenagers, adults abovc forty years of age and very old people. In order to feel comfortable and active or energetic throughout the year, seasonal variations should also be carried out in the diet.

So we see that diet is an integral part of one's life. After all, "a man is what he eats"!

How to Lose Weight

It is sometimes of interest to make a check on how many calories one is taking daily, but it is usually not necessary because the body weight constitutes an unerring index of whether the food is furnishing energy equal to, in excess of, or below the energy requirements of the body. When the energy intake just about balances the energy expenditure, the body neither gains nor loses weight. Minor weight variations (½-1 kg) from day-to-day are of little significance and often may be due to fluctuations in water content of the body. If the body weight is stagnant over a considerable period of time, it means that the energy value of the food intake is adjusted naturally so that it is practically equal to the energy requirement.

After an adult has attained full growth, it is advantageous to maintain the body weight at about a certain norm for the height. Being overweight or underweight represent disadvantages which usually result in lesser efficiency or poorer health.

If the body weight is persistently, though slowly, increasing, there is certainty that the energy value of the food intake is greater than the energy needs of the body. Even a small excess such as 150-200 calories per day (equivalent to 2 teaspoons of butter or 300-400 ml of any aerated drink), if persistently indulged in, will mean the storage of 8-10 kg of body fat in a year's time! Usually overeating of calories is the result of too great a fondness for high-calorie foods (fried foods, sweets and starchy foods). Decreased muscular activity is also often a contributing factor; for instance, the sedentary nature of office work, commuting by scooters and cars, etc. As one becomes older, there is a tendency for both the basal metabolism (energy for internal body functions) and the physical activity to be lessened.

If one carries over into later life the food habits of younger years, the weight is almost certain to increase undesirably. Then it will be necessary to take either less food or more exercise, or both, in order to bring the weight down to about the normal for age 30. A decrease in food intake of 500 calories daily below the amount that would presumably keep the body weight constant, will normally result in 'burning' or melting of fatty tissues of the body to an extent that will reduce the body weight by ½ kg per week. The maximum weight reduction considered safe is 1 kg per week, which is 1,000 calories per day.

Obesity is certainly not desirable, as it leads to inconvenience in moving about, embarrassment, inefficiency and lack of ambition. Obesity also results in diseases of the heart, circulatory system, kidneys and pancreas and lessened chances of

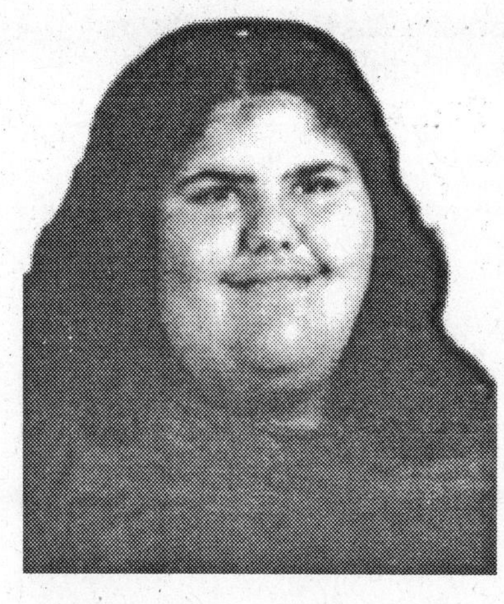

long life. It is prone to develop at 34-45 years of age and is especially disadvantageous after 50 years of age. The dangers of overweight are naturally increased with a larger excess of weight and advancing years. For instance, between 40 and 44 years, a 20 per cent excess over normal weight means 30-40 per cent mortality above the normal for that age bracket. A 40 per cent excess of weight involves an 80-100 per cent increase in mortality rate. To put it more simply, a 50-year-old man, who is 25 kg overweight, has about half the life expectancy of one of the same age who is of normal weight. For younger adults, a moderate amount of extra weight may be acceptable but after 40, a moderate amount of leanness tends to promote longevity.

Diet

For the ordinary overweight individual, by far the most satisfactory way to effect weight reduction is simply to cut down sharply on concentrated energy foods (sugar, starch and fats), keeping on with an otherwise well balanced and adequate diet. Such a diet does not involve actually going hungry and it can be maintained over fairly long periods without causing any harm. By adding limited amounts of high-calorie foods, this diet

Calorie Content of Common Raw Food Items in Convenient Measures

Item	*Measure*	*Weight (Grams)*	*Energy (Calories)*
Cereals			
Rice	1 Cup (small)	150	520
Wheat flour	"	90	310
Millet flour	"	90	300
Pulses			
Bengal gram	"	130	485
Other dals	"	135	460
Whole pulses			
Green gram	"	140	470
Cowpea (lobia)	"	135	440
Rajma	"	120	415
Soyabean	"	130	530
Green leafy vegetables	5 Bundles	100	62
Other vegetables	—	100	105
Nuts and oilseeds			
Almonds	10 nos.	15	85
Cashewnuts	10 nos.	15	95
Coconut (fresh)	1 no.	115	510
Coconut (dry)	½ no.	45	290
Groundnuts	50 nos.	15	85
Sesame seeds	1 tsp.	3	15
Oils/Vanaspati ghee	2 tsp.	10 ml.	100
Spices			
Chilli powder	1 tsp.	7	17
Coriander seeds	1 tsp.	7	20
Cumin seeds	1 tsp.	5	18
Fenugreek (Methi)	1 tsp.	6	20
Mustard seeds	1 tsp.	10	5
Garlic	7 pods	3	4
Onion	1 med.	50	30
Animal foods			
Egg (hen)	One	60	100
Mutton	—	100	194
Fish (lean)	—	100	100
Fish (fatty)	—	100	150

Notes:* *tsp *= teaspoon (5 ml.),* ***tbsp*** *= tablespoon (15 ml.),* ***1 cup (small)*** *= 150 ml.*

can be continued into the post-reduction period in order to maintain the desired body weight. Such a reducing diet should be based on one's food preferences so that it can be used indefinitely.

The reducing diet should be built around certain basic foods, which provide the nutritive essentials, like the protein-rich foods (*dals*, meat, egg, milk) and fruits and vegetables to provide minerals and vitamins. Certain foods, like sugar and fats, chiefly provide calories and no other nutritive essentials. Varying the amount of these foods is the easiest way to alter the caloric intake without affecting the other nutritive values of the diet.

Other foods that are useful mainly for their energy value and carry only minor amounts of other nutrients are sweets (jam, jelly, desserts), starchy foods (bread, breakfast cereals, cereal puddings) and fatty foods (fatty meats, salad dressings, chocolates, cream). Another way to cut down on calories is to eat foods in their natural state, unadulterated by added calories in the form of sugar or fat. A medium-sized apple furnishes 70-80 calories, a baked apple 210 calories and a piece of apple pie about 370 calories.

It should be emphasised that while it is entirely possible to get all the required nutrients in a well-planned reducing diet, supplementary vitamins and minerals may well be a safeguard for persons on drastic or lengthy reducing regimens. This is especially true of the fat-soluble vitamins (A, D, E, K), since fats are sharply curtailed, and many people cannot take large amounts of leafy vegetables.

Controlling Body Weight

The best first step to prevent overweight is to check the increase immediately by making changes in the diet related to the activity. Instead of reducing the total food intake, it is much better to adjust it according to the energy expenditure.

It is convenient to consider the energy expenditure of people employed in an urban society as divided into three parts corresponding to three eight-hour periods. One part is spent in bed, the second at work and travelling to work, and the third in various non-occupational activities and recreation. The rate of energy expenditure when in bed approximates 400-500 calories per 8 hours. At work the energy expenditure is determined by the nature of the occupation. In a sedentary job it amounts to about 900 calories per 8 hours; in a job involving moderate physical activity, to about 1,200 calories per 8 hours. On an average 900 calories per 8 hours can be considered as the expenditure for non-occupational activity.

Based on the above classification, the total food intake can also be divided into three — breakfast, lunch and dinner. Breakfast is our first meal and comes just before the 8-hour period of work requiring maximum energy. Thus, it should be our heaviest meal providing us the maximum calories. The main activity after lunch is non-occupational and recreational apart from some portion left over from the work period. This implies that lunch should be lighter than breakfast. The 8-hour period of rest in bed follows dinner, which should be the lightest meal in terms of energy value, as this rest period involves the minimum energy expenditure.

Daily Calorie Requirement	
Age	*Calorie Requirement*
1. Up to 6 months	120 calories per kg. body weight
2. 7-12 months	100 " "
3. 1-3 years	1200 calories (for full body weight)
4. 4-6 years	1500 " "
5. 7-9 years	1800 " "
6. 10-12 years	2100 " "
7. 13-15 years (boys)	2500 " "
8. 13-15 years (girls)	2200 " "
9. 16-18 years (boys)	3000 " "
10. 16-18 years (girls)	2200 " "
11. Men a) Light work b) Medium work c) Heavy work	 2200 " " 2800 " " 3400 " "
12. Women a) Light work b) Medium work c) Heavy work	 1900 " " 2200 " " 2800 " "

Notes:

1. *Calorie requirements depend upon the body weight, occupation and age of the persons. The calorie requirements given above are average figures for medium-weight persons.*

2. *For older persons, reduce the calorie requirement as follows:*

   40-49 years — 5%

   50-59 years — 10%

   60-69 years — 20%

   Over 70 years — 30%

This diet plan is known as the 'breakfast diet' plan, since breakfast is the heaviest and most important of all meals, according to this plan.

Taking a heavy breakfast, a lighter lunch and the lightest possible dinner prove to be an effective check on body weight and an easy way to shed the extra kilos without cutting down on the total dietary intake.

Quick-reducing Gimmicks

Probably no type of quackery is more profitable at present than the special remedies sold to effect weight reduction, and the various adjuncts supposed to make weight loss easy and safe. They flourish because people have become conscious of the need to do something about the problem of overweight, but still hope to do it as painlessly as possible. So they are credulous about remedies that promise "you can eat all you want and still lose weight"!

Reducing diets, fast becoming a fad now, are being religiously propagated by various so-called health and beauty experts and clinics. How effective are they? These reducing schemes are among the many offenders of good health. They win favour with overweight people simply because reducing is difficult. The only way a fat person can become slim and stay slim is by decreasing his intake of calories and increasing his exercise — not temporarily, but permanently. This takes more will power and tenacity than many fat persons can muster. So they snatch at any promise of assistance, whether it comes from pills, unusual diets or special eating schedules.

A popular remedy for weight reduction is a fixed diet plan. A lot of magazines and books have been carrying these planned diets, with menus for a whole week or even a month. It seems remarkable that people would be so eager to follow menu plans made out by someone who cannot know their food preferences or circumstances, or the availability of various food items at different times. Either they must believe that the diet has some magical properties, or they simply want someone else to do all the thinking for them.

Then there are also the peculiar diets based on only a few foods, such as the all-fruit diet, the green vegetables diet, the milk-banana diet, the raw egg and orange juice diet, the raw tomato and boiled egg diet etc. These appeal to some people either as short cuts in reducing or by their sheer unusualness. Such diets are not only monotonous to take, but also so one-sided that they are sure to be too low and too high in some of the nutrients.

These reducing diets can often help reduce weight, but they rarely provide a lasting solution to obesity. Often the drastic weight-reducing diet is so monotonous that it usually defeats its purpose. The reducer becomes so hungry for normal food that he may use up a week's allotment of calories in a one-hour eating orgy. A similar fate awaits those who try to lose weight by skipping meals — they often eat so much at their meals that they gain instead of losing weight!

Some people believe that toasting bread lowers its calorie content. It does not — the application of heat causes a chemical alteration of the starch, but does not make it any less fattening. Washing cooked rice is another trick that is supposed to help dieters — it simply washes away the water-soluble vitamins, not the calories.

Reducing pills too do not have a lasting effect. The 'filler' (a chemically inactive substance like methyl cellulose, which is not absorbed by the body) gives a sensation of fullness and temporarily lessens hunger pangs. However, its efficacy lasts only so long as the dieter manages to exercise restraint at his next meal.

A purpose somehow similar to that of the filler is served by another drug, the 'depressant', usually an active chemical like amphetamine, which interferes with the appetite-controlling centre of the brain to reduce the dieter's desire to eat.

One drug that really melts fat is the 'stimulator', most often a thyroid extract. This acts as a sort of chemical exerciser, speeding up the body's reactions so that the calories are consumed faster than usual.

Another type of pill reduces weight without really affecting obesity. This is the 'diuretic', a dehydrating agent that stimulates the kidneys to drain out water from the body tissues. The loss is not in the fat at all, only in water. The pill-taker may fool the weighing machine, but not his tailor!

One of these drugs is sometimes prescribed by a physician as a morale booster — they help induce a weight loss that encourages the struggling reducer to stick to his slimming programme a little longer. But many of them cause undesirable side-effects such as nervousness and insomnia. To reduce, the patient must still restrict his intake of calories and increase his exercise. When he does so with the help of synthetic appetite curbers or stimulants, he achieves nothing towards the development of sensible permanent eating and exercise habits. Almost invariably he will regain the lost weight (and frequently more) shortly after he stops taking the drugs.

So you see there is no short cut to reducing!

How to Gain Weight

It is not necessary that a diet be prescribed for the obese only. Many people are underweight too. Due to the lack of correct dietary advice they attribute their lean and thin figure to heredity. The problem of being underweight is very typical in young people. The nutritional requirement in adolescents is conditioned primarily by the spurt of growth that occurs at puberty. There is an increased demand for calories and protein at that time.

The increased caloric need is ordinarily reflected in the appetite. Unless additional food is provided at mealtime, the individual makes it up by eating in between meals. This habit leads to an intake of an unbalanced diet and results in slowing down normal growth.

Failure to meet the additional requirement for the body-building proteins at this time is believed to be an important cause of very slow height gain, loss of resistance to diseases, hair loss and skin problems. So certain dietary modifications are necessary.

Standard Heights and Weights for Men and Women (Medium Frame) (For 25 years and above)

Height		Weight (Kg.)
Cms.	*Ft.*	
MEN		
157	5' 2"	56.3-60.3
160	5' 3"	57.6-61.7
162	5' 4"	58.9-63.5
165	5' 5"	60.8-65.3
168	5' 6"	62.2-66.7
170	5' 7"	64.0-68.5
173	5' 8"	65.8-70.8
175	5' 9"	67.6-72.6
178	5' 10"	69.4-74.4
180	5' 11"	71.2-76.2
183	6' 0"	73.0-78.5
185	6' 1"	75.3-80.7
188	6' 2"	77.6-83.5
190	6' 3"	79.8-85.9
WOMEN		
152	5' 0"	50.8-54.4
155	5' 1"	51.7-55.3
157	5' 2"	53.1-56-7
160	5' 3"	54.4-58.1
162	5' 4"	56.3-59.9
165	5' 5"	57.6-61.2
168	5' 6"	58.9-63.5
170	5' 7"	60.8-65.3
173	5' 8"	62.2-66.7
175	5' 9"	64.0-68.5
178	5' 10"	65.8-70.3
180	5' 11"	67.1-71.7
183	6' 0"	68.5-73.9

Diet

For increasing body weight, the total calorie intake should be in excess of the energy requirement.

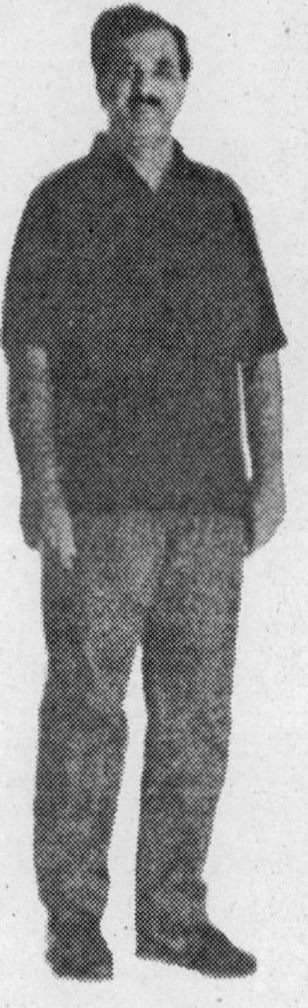

If about 500 calories per day were taken in excess of the regular diet, there would be a weekly gain of about half a kilogram in the weight of the individual. These calories can be in the form of four bananas, or 100 gm peanuts, or 250 gm fresh dates or half a kilogram mangoes, etc.

A liberal supply of protein is necessary for tissue building. So protein-rich foods like milk products, meat, fish, poultry, eggs, all *dals*, peanuts etc. should be taken as much as possible.

High-calorie fatty foods such as nuts and dried fruits, cream, butter, *ghee*, vanaspati and oils help to increase body weight. But fatty foods should not be taken at the beginning of a meal as they reduce the appetite.

Leafy vegetables, with low carbohydrate content, should be restricted and preference given to those with a high-calorie equivalent — like potatoes and yam, cereals and cereal products such as bread, biscuits etc. These are a storehouse of calories and proteins, hence should be taken liberally.

With such a liberal diet, there is no necessity for extra vitamin and mineral supplements. A glass of mixed fruit juice or a bowl of mixed vegetable soup or a plate of fresh fruits/vegetable salad or *chaat* will provide the necessary vitamins and minerals. Liquids, especially water, should not be taken before or with the meal, but only after the meal, so that the food intake is not reduced.

Regular outdoor exercise (in the morning) helps to stimulate the appetite. Constipation may reduce the appetite, so bowel movements should be regulated by a judicious intake of fluids, fresh fruits and vegetables, and exercise.

Whatever you may eat during the day (following the above diet advice), make sure to have a heavy dinner. Top this with a glass of milk at bedtime. No after-dinner walks for the underweight.

If an undernourished adolescent follows such a dietary regime, the body will pick up growth, and a marked increase in the height and weight will be seen. Once the growth period of adolescence has passed, then by following the above plan, weight would only be increased.

Anaemia

Anaemia is a condition characterised by too little haemoglobin or too few red blood cells in the blood. It is considered a symptom of an underlying disease or condition rather than a disease itself.

Anaemia gives rise to the same general symptoms whatever the cause. A person leading a sedentary life may have a moderate degree of anaemia and yet be free of symptoms, though these develop if unaccustomed exercise is done. A degree of anaemia is always associated with an inability to make sustained physical effort. As anaemia often develops very slowly, the patient may gradually, unconsciously reduce physical activity to a lower level. It is not unusual to find anaemic women doing all the normal household chores, but slowly.

Common symptoms are: skin pallor, fatigue, weakness, fainting spells, breathlessness on exertion, palpitations, or increased awareness of your heartbeat, sore mouth or tongue, headache, lack of appetite, loss of hair and tingling in hands and feet.

There are three main causes of anaemia:

- Loss of blood due to external (injury, bleeding piles, excessive menstruation) or internal (gastrointestinal: common causes being medications such as aspirin and ibuprofen, and cancer) bleeding;

- Haemolysis, i.e., increased destruction of blood cells, which may be due to the defect in the red blood cells or the circulating haemolytic agents;

- Reduced or insufficient production of red blood cells, which may be due to an inadequate intake, absorption or utilisation of factors essential for blood formation.

The life of the red blood cells is 120 days and the bone marrow replaces them at a rate which enables their number to be maintained. For the production of red blood cells, many nutrients are needed. The most important of them being iron, vitamin B_{12} and folic acid.

It is unusual for anaemia to occur in a healthy person solely as a direct result of a poor diet. However the diet may have insufficient nutrients to meet the increased needs of a chronic problem. Disorders of the digestive system may also lead to impaired absorption of the essential nutrients resulting in anaemia.

The most common variety of anaemia throughout the world is the iron-deficiency anaemia. It mostly affects women in their reproductive years, infants and children.

Anaemia occurs when there is too little iron stored in the body. Young children and adults may not get enough absorbable iron in the foods they eat, which can lead to anaemia. The digestive system may not be able to absorb enough iron, or a person may become anaemic through excessive loss of blood; this can affect women with heavy menstrual periods, and people with stomach or duodenal ulcers, haemorrhoids or piles, or even hookworm infection.

Iron intake may be adequate in a diet consisting of cereals as a staple; the problem is that usually only 10 per cent of the ingested iron is absorbed. This is because, the cereals, besides having a high iron content are also rich in phytates, which inhibit iron absorption. This problem is corrected by increasing the calcium content of the diet, by eating curds (or any other milk product) with the meals. Eating betel leaf (*paan*) with lime (*choona*) after a meal also helps in providing calcium. Insufficient intake of vitamin C is also a factor in the poor absorption of iron by the body. The age-old practice of squeezing lemon (*nimbu*) juice on the food and salads is a way of correcting this problem and thus enhancing the iron absorption.

Sweat also contains iron, therefore people living in hot conditions suffer from iron-deficiency more than their counterparts living in cooler areas.

If you suspect that you have anaemia, it is important to visit your doctor. Anaemia can weaken the body's resistance to illness, and limits the energy and productivity levels. It can also indicate a more serious medical condition. It is important, therefore, to discover and treat the cause of anaemia.

Diet

- Make sure you include plenty of green, leafy vegetables in your diet: cooked, raw as salads or chutneys.
- Iron-fortified foods, like many breakfast cereals, can also boost iron reserves.
- Avoid caffeinated drinks — coffee, tea, and colas — during meals because they interfere with iron absorption.
- If you are a woman with heavy periods or if you are pregnant, talk to your doctor about taking an iron supplement.
- Use an iron pot or *karahi* when cooking. Some iron from the pot will be incorporated into the food that is being cooked in it.

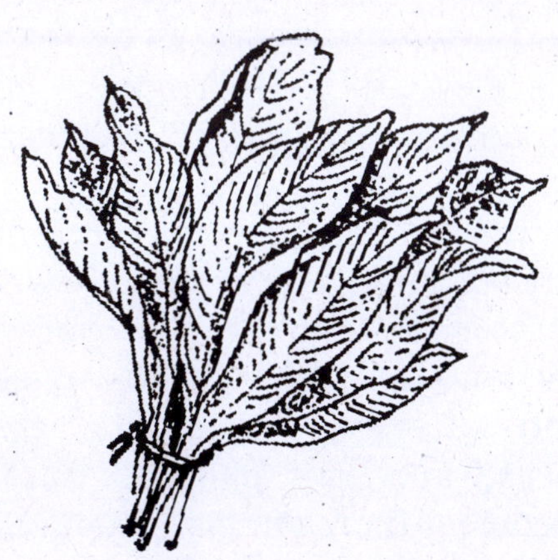

Allergies

Food allergy has always been a highly topical subject featuring regularly in medical journals. Food intolerance or allergy denotes a reproducible clinical reaction to food. It must be distinguished from food aversions, which comprise psychological avoidance and intolerance, where the clinical response does not occur when the food is given in a disguised form. Not all people who believe they are sensitive to a particular food really are. They may in fact dislike the food, or they may have eaten it coincidentally with the onset of an illness and thereby developed a psychological intolerance.

Food allergies are more common in infants and young children (10-15% of children suffer from symptoms due to food intolerance). Cow's milk protein intolerance, the most common food allergy in childhood, has a prevalence between 5% and 7.5%. After the age of five years, there is a tendency for the spontaneous disappearance of the food allergy, while allergy to inhaled substances, such as pollens, dust and animal hair, becomes increasingly frequent.

The list of foods that are claimed to cause allergic reactions is very large. It includes such diverse items like eggs, milk, wheat, fish (especially shellfish and other sea foods), various meats, nuts, mustard, tomatoes, oranges and chocolates!

Allergic reactions may affect any system of the body, producing various symptoms. For example, the skin may show a rash, eczema or swollen patches. The respiratory system may be involved in bronchial asthma, sinusitis or bronchitis. The digestive system may show indigestion, vomiting, abdominal pain, diarrhoea and failure of normal growth.

The other allergic symptoms are headache, swelling of joints, conjunctivitis, swelling of lips and tongue, etc. The claims that allergy may be involved in migraine and epilepsy still require confirmation, though a minority of sufferers from migraine are able to incriminate particular foods, like cheese, chocolate, citrus fruits, and alcoholic drinks as provoking agents. Similarly, hyperactivity in children (usually boys) being aggravated by some artificial food colours is also a subject of controversy.

There are other more specific examples of food sensitivity, the most important of which is coeliac disease or gluten enteropathy. There is malabsorption, weight loss, impaired growth in children, and other manifestations of malnutrition. Coeliac disease is due to atrophy (flattening of the cells) of the inner lining of the small intestine. In this disease, a fraction of wheat, the gluten, acts as the allergen. When wheat is completely eliminated from the diet, patients recover.

One has to be very careful in diagnosing the exact allergen — that is, the food responsible for the causation of allergy symptoms.

In some cases of food allergy, the symptoms develop rapidly and dramatically, almost immediately after eating the offending food, and the diagnosis is easy to make. There are some people, for instance, whose lips swell the moment their mouth touches a peanut, and if by chance they swallow some they will have several systemic symptoms — vomiting, rash, even asthma. More often, it is not so easy to associate symptoms with any particular food, especially if there is a delay of some hours between the eating of the suspected food and the onset of illness. If the symptoms are chronic or recur frequently, they should disappear on a diet (elimination diet) of very few foods (rice, carrots, lettuce, refined oil, sugar, and water) that do not cause food sensitivity. Suspected foods then can be re-introduced one at a time. Skin tests are not very reliable.

It is also observed that people tend to outgrow their allergies. Foods known to have caused reactions in childhood may be tried years later with no reactions at all. All people with a well-defined allergy should know about it and inform their doctor. Otherwise they may suffer a severe or even a fatal reaction from a therapeutic injection given for the treatment of some other disease! For instance, a person sensitive to eggs may react badly to immunising injections prepared on an egg medium, such as those for polio or influenza.

Diet

The diet prescription for an allergic person must be specific, individually modified and adjusted, according to the cause of the food allergy.

If the causative food factor is identified, then it can be totally eliminated from the diet, and the symptoms would not recur. For example, if the responsible article of food is one that is not consumed regularly (like shellfish), then it can easily be avoided. It is far more difficult in the case of eggs, milk and wheat, which are present in so many foods — cakes, sauces, soups, biscuits, bread, pasta etc.

Substitution of an alternative food may be possible in the case of milk allergy. A person sensitive to cow's milk may not necessarily be sensitive to goat's milk. Soybean milk or groundnut milk can also be used as substitutes. Similarly, one sensitive to wheat may do well on oats, rice, barley or corn.

Heating the food may change its properties regarding the causation of allergic symptoms. A person sensitive to raw milk or lightly boiled eggs may be able to tolerate boiled milk or hard-boiled eggs. Many times persons sensitive to eggs are able to take the yolks (yellow part) especially if well cooked, although the egg white continues to cause symptoms.

It is not really difficult to live with a food allergy — you just have to be a little extra careful!

Dental Health

Good teeth and gums are important for maintaining health and in promoting good digestion. Furthermore, the appearance of bad teeth is undesirable for aesthetic reasons too. Diet has a major role to play in dental health. Dietary factors and disease-causing bacteria are primarily responsible for dental diseases.

During the development of teeth, a protein base is formed and this subsequently gets deposited with minerals. During this process a variety of nutrients including vitamin D, calcium and phosphorus must be present in required quantities to ensure proper calcification.

Enamel is to teeth what skin is to the body and serves as a protective barrier. Under-nutrition during early life can affect the development of teeth, and particularly the enamel. There can be pitting, furrowing or even absence of enamel depending on the severity of malnutrition. Since enamel has no mechanism to repair itself, malnutrition during tooth development produces a permanent defect in the enamel. This also reduces the resistance of teeth to infections.

The foundations of the first teeth are laid down before birth. If the diet of a pregnant woman lacks adequate protein, vitamins and minerals, the baby's teeth erupt late and lack the desired hardness. Several vitamin deficiencies, especially of vitamins A, D and C, have been shown to lead to dental abnormalities.

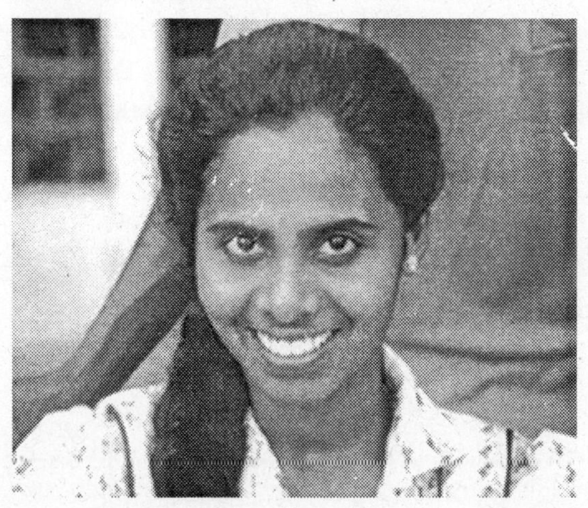

Vitamin A deficiency, apart from affecting the eyes, also leads to inadequate bone growth resulting in a defective alignment and formation of teeth. Vitamin A is also needed to keep the enamel healthy.

Vitamin C is required for healthy gums and its deficiency results in swollen and bleeding gums. Such weak and unhealthy gums cannot firmly hold the teeth.

Vitamin D is necessary for absorption of calcium from the intestine. Deficiency of either vitamin D or calcium can result in the pitting of teeth. In order to get these vitamins and minerals, a liberal intake of fresh fruits and vegetables, especially green leafy vegetables, red and yellow vegetables and fruits, citrus fruits, milk and milk products should be encouraged.

Among dental diseases, dental caries or tooth decay continues to be a major problem — mostly afflicting children, since newly-erupted teeth are more susceptible to decay and young children do not brush their teeth properly. They also eat and drink more frequently than adults. Carbohydrates, especially refined, and simple sugars, which promote the growth of bacteria, are mainly responsible for caries. It also results from frequent consumption of sticky or adhesive forms of sugar-containing foods such as chocolates and toffees, particularly between meals. These sticky foods remain as tiny particles in the mouth and produce certain acids, which damage the teeth.

Another common dental disease is the periodontal disease or pyorrhoea. In this disease the gums are affected. A soft diet, rich in carbohydrates that stick around the teeth, forms a good medium for the growth of bacteria. Bacteria can seep down beneath the gum margins and damage the underlying tissues and bone supporting the teeth. Vitamin C deficiency may exaggerate these symptoms.

Milk sugars, if allowed to come in contact with the teeth for long, can produce dental decay. A feeding bottle kept in the mouth of infants throughout the night during sleep can result in 'nursing bottle syndrome', which leads to extensive decay of teeth. Hence, after milk is consumed, gargling or rinsing of mouth with water is advised.

There are many minerals in drinking water. Of these, fluorine is an important mineral with respect to dental disease. A concentration of fluoride in drinking water between 0.5 and 1 parts per million (ppm) protects against caries, but if it exceeds 2 ppm mottling of teeth occurs. If the fluoride content of water is less than 0.5 ppm, the prevalence of caries goes up. A fluoride intake of one to three milligrams per day (as with fluoridated drinking water) increases the enamel's resistance to acid attack, especially if the fluoride is taken while the tooth's enamel is being formed in the jaws before the permanent teeth erupt.

Diet

Excessive use of irritants like betel leaves (*paan*), betel nuts, tobacco, spices, alcohol, very hot foodstuffs and smoking is found to cause oral cancers. But then, excess of every thing seems to cause some or the other sort of cancer.

Anything that is hard and fibrous in nature is beneficial to dental health, since it exercises the teeth and also keeps them clean. Hence, children should be encouraged to eat sugarcane, guava, or carrot, which have the above properties and in addition provide good nutrients. Eating sticky sweets, jams, jellies or soft starchy foods between meals should be discouraged. Keeping the gums and teeth clean by gargling and rinsing the mouth properly with water after eating anything and brushing the teeth properly in the morning and after dinner is necessary to maintain dental health. A regular dental check-up is always beneficial.

Diabetes

Diabetes mellitus is a syndrome characterised by a raised glucose concentration in the blood, due to the deficiency or diminished effectiveness of insulin. (Insulin is produced in our body by a gland known as the pancreas.) The condition shows itself by symptoms like excessive thirst, excessive urination, excessive hunger, unexplained weight-loss, failing eyesight and repeated infections.

There are two basic types of diabetes: insulin-dependent and non-insulin-dependent. Insulin-dependent, also known as juvenile diabetes, usually starts in younger people; their pancreas secrete little or no insulin and they must receive one or more injections of insulin each day to control their blood glucose.

Non-insulin-dependent diabetes, also known as maturity-onset diabetes, is the more common type, usually starting in middle age; the patient's pancreas secrete normal amounts of insulin, but it is ineffective and the response of blood glucose to insulin is subnormal. This type of diabetes is closely linked to obesity. It has also been found that a diet high in fat is likely to lead to diabetes. When people with a family history of diabetes are obese, the incidence of their becoming diabetic (in later life) is over 50 per cent. In females, the risk of diabetes depends on whether they have put on weight on the upper part of the body or the lower. There is an increased risk of diabetes for women who have put on weight in the neck, shoulders and abdominal regions. Women who have put on weight on the thighs and hips are relatively safer.

In a study conducted on 3,000 significantly overweight participants having pronounced 'impaired glucose tolerance' (meaning a high but not yet diabetic blood sugar level), a low-fat diet combined with moderate exercise dramatically reduced maturity-onset diabetes risk. It was found that the diet-exercise programme cut diabetes risk by 58%, especially among people of age 60 and older. The average age of people in the study was 51, although ages ranged from 25 to 85. They were put on a low-fat diet and told to engage in moderate physical exercise, such as walking for 30 minutes. The diet was centred on lowering the fat intake to less than 25% of overall calories. Not only did making the lifestyle changes reduce their risk of getting diabetes, but these individuals also lost 5%-7% of their body weight. Scientists believe that weight loss lowers diabetes risk by helping muscle cells to handle blood sugar more efficiently.

Eating the right diet helps avoid having to live with diabetes in the future. In a landmark study, over 42,000 men, 40 to 75 years of age, were studied to see which men developed diabetes over the next 12 years. More than 1,300 men developed diabetes. But this was most commonly seen in men who ate a 'western' diet, which is, higher amounts of red meat, processed meat, french fries, high-fat dairy products, refined cereals and pulses, and sweets and desserts. Men who ate a diet of more vegetables, fruit, fish, poultry, and whole grains were less likely to get diabetes. In men who ate a predominantly western diet, the risk of diabetes went up even more if they didn't exercise or were overweight.

The rising frequency of obesity was thought to be one of the main reasons for the problem. But this study showed that it might be only one factor. Even men who were not overweight and ate a western diet were more likely to get diabetes.

Diet

Diet appears to be an essential part of diabetic treatment, since a large proportion of patients with maturity-onset diabetes are obese.

The most important dietary measure for the obese diabetics is the restriction of caloric intake to reduce their body weight to that of normal adults of the same sex and height. The caloric requirement of an elderly, obese, diabetic patient lies between 1,000 and 1,600 calories. Weight reduction should be gradual, usually not more than 2 kg per month, which corresponds to a deficit of 500 calories per day. Achievement of the desirable weight is almost always associated with better control of blood glucose level. Sometimes weight control through dietary restriction can control diabetes too, without any help from pills or insulin. Regular exercise is important, as it is effective in controlling weight.

Ideally, an elderly diabetic patient of normal body weight should consume 1,400 to 1,800 calories per day.

In the case of young, active diabetics, under-nutrition is undesirable. It should be avoided, as it would affect the growth pattern of the person. The caloric requirement in this case would lie between 1,800 and 3,000 calories. However, care should be taken to avoid obesity.

Large individual loads of carbohydrates or starch are discouraged, especially when they include concentrated and refined carbohydrates, sugar in particular. For example, a bowl of *kheer*, a pastry, or a plate of *aloo bonda* in one serving would be considered as a concentrated source of carbohydrate. The quantities of such items per serving should be reduced, not because they are harmful to diabetics (they are not!) – these items tend to increase the total caloric intake of the person.

A diabetic has to keep a check on his weight through his caloric intake. The best way to cut down on calories is to cut down on sugars (sweets and aerated drinks are high sources of calories) and fats (fried foods, nuts, dried fruits, pickles-in-oil are high sources of calories).

Levels of cholesterol tend to be higher in diabetics (after the age of 40 years) than in non-diabetics of the same age. This is associated with a high incidence of coronary heart disease. So the use of saturated fat is discouraged. The proportion of fat may be manipulated by limiting eggs (especially egg yolks) to no more than 3 per week, by replacing, as much as possible, whole milk and processed cheese with skimmed milk and cottage cheese (*paneer*) respectively, mutton and other red meats with fish and chicken (white meats), and by replacing butter, cream, *ghee* and *vanaspati* with polyunsaturated oils, like *til* oil, mustard oil, groundnut oil and so on.

The fibre content of the diet should be increased as much as possible, as it lowers the absorption of glucose and cholesterol from the diet. Whole grain flour and whole pulses should be preferred in the diet instead of refined flour and washed pulses. (Do not throw away the *chokar* from the *atta.*) Wherever possible, fruits and vegetables should not be peeled.

In diabetes, there is no medical objection to taking alcoholic drinks in moderation, provided the patient realises that he must take account of their caloric values (whisky, gin, etc. contain about 70 calories per 30 ml.). Diabetics are particularly prone to having fatty liver. Even the slightest sign of impaired liver function is a strict contra-indication for alcohol.

In general, a diabetic patient needs a normal, balanced, high-fibre diet, strict weight control (by controlling the calories), exercise and extremely moderate use of alcoholic beverages, together with medication (if required).

Gout

Gout is an inherited disease mostly occurring in males and is due to an abnormal uric acid metabolism. The uric acid level in the blood is high and there is deposition of uric acid salts in the cartilages (soft bones) of the joints. There are recurrent attacks of pain and swelling of the joints, frequently the joint of the big toe, but other joints may also be affected. Only 5-10 per cent of women suffer from gout. In such cases gout seldom manifests before menopause. The incidence of kidney diseases in gouty patients is very high. Kidney stones in gouty patients and members of their family are also a common occurrence. The stones are mostly of uric acid.

Diet

The source of uric acid is food with a high purine content such as meat, especially glandular meat like liver, pancreas and kidney, fish like herring, salmon and sardine. Anyone with a family history of gout should avoid these at all times.

Foods of moderate purine content like meat (other than glandular), chicken, lobster, prawn, fish like pomfret, vegetables like brinjal, cauliflower, spinach, peas and all kinds of beans, asparagus, mushrooms, all *dals*, fruits like *chickoo* and custard apple should be avoided during a gouty attack. They should be taken in moderation otherwise.

All cereals, milk and milk products, eggs, sugar and sweets, fruits and vegetables other than the ones mentioned above can be consumed liberally at all times.

Obese persons are more prone to gout. The body weight should be reduced to normal not only to prevent recurrence of gout but also to prevent changes in the weight-bearing joints that occur in the obese.

Fat consumption should be restricted partly because its ingestion tends to cause retention of urates by the kidney, and partly to prevent obesity.

During an attack of gout the main source of energy should be from carbohydrates for its 'protein sparing effect', which reduces the endogenous protein breakdown.

Liberal fluids should be taken to ensure a daily excretion of about 2,000 ml of urine. Tea and coffee do contain purines, but they are not converted by the body into uric acid. So, about 2 or 3 cups a day are permitted.

Usually, gouty patients tolerate white wine or whisky, but not beer or red wines.

Fever

Fever is not a disease. It is a symptom. When any bacterial or viral infection enters our body, it puts up its defence. In such a situation, the temperature of our body rises. This we call fever. There is a breakdown of the body protein and loss of other nutrients as well. For this reason, and because there is usually a loss of appetite and consequent diminished food intake, a person having fever loses weight; and if the fever is prolonged, he may even become severely emaciated. With fever there is also an increased amount of excretion of vitamins B complex and C, through urine.

In any kind of fever, an effort should be made to prevent the undue loss of body protein by taking a diet in which the protein content is in excess of the normal requirement. There is no ground for the old belief that a high protein intake increases the fever, nor is it right to follow the old saying, 'feed the cold and starve the fever'.

Diet management in fever is made more difficult by the loss of appetite associated with most fevers, and it may be further complicated by the presence of nausea. Much can be done to help by ensuring that the patient's mouth is kept clean. If the tongue is furred, it should not be surprising that the patient has distaste for food.

Using a mouthwash before and after each meal would be of great help. Fresh cucumber or tomato with a little salt, pepper and limejuice is a good appetiser.

Diet

In short-duration fevers such as influenza, pneumonia, typhoid and malaria that last for just a few days, not weeks, the diet's chief objective is to save the patient from all possible exertion, even in his food intake. So, for the first two or three days, the diet should be fluid or semi-fluid. For example, milk flavoured with chocolate, coffee or tea or given as eggnog or milk shakes, custards, soups, fruit juices etc. It is important that the liquid intake of the patient be at least two to three litres in a day.

As soon as the temperature falls, and the patient's appetite improves, he can gradually be put on a soft, and then a normal, diet.

In long-duration fever, that is, fever exceeding seven days (as in tuberculosis), it is necessary to see that the dietary intake, and particularly the intake of protein and energy, is sufficient to meet the extra requirements imposed by fever.

The diet should have high-energy (calorie) value, up to fifty per cent more than the normal intake. These calories can be obtained by giving cream in the form of fruit cream or as a topping in other desserts, adding glucose to fruit juices, and butter in soups.

A liberal protein intake is necessary to make good the loss of body protein. This can be done by ensuring that every meal includes a protein dish in the form of milk desserts, egg or *paneer* preparations, *dal* soups, curd preparations etc. The food should be soft, easily digestible, well cooked and appetising. No large meals please! Six small meals are preferable to three large ones.

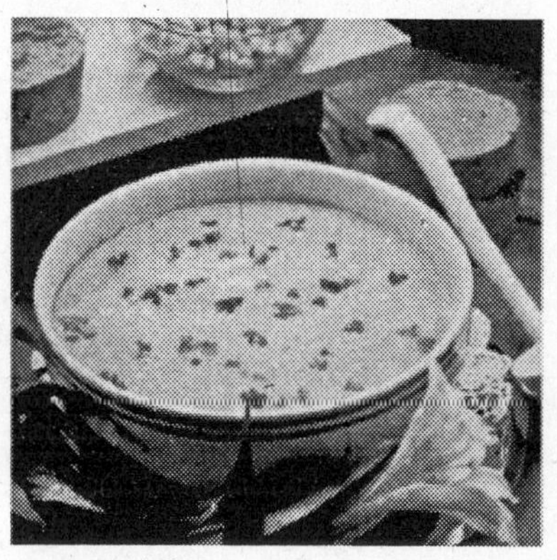

Owing to the loss of water through increased sweating in fever, the fluid intake should also be increased to two-and-a-half to three litres. Apart from water, salt is also lost in sweat, and this loss can be rectified by taking salt in limejuice, fruit juices and soups. The vitamin losses incurred through urine, in a febrile state, can be made good with the help of fresh fruit juices and vegetable soups.

On following these diet suggestions, one will find that the associated weakness with fever is much less and recovery speedier.

Common Gastric Problems

IRRITABLE BOWEL SYNDROME

Nervous diarrhoea, spastic constipation and acute pain in the lower abdomen are common symptoms of irritable bowel syndrome. The disorder is often stress-related. Although there is no cure for this disorder as yet, careful attention to diet and stress management helps keep symptoms under control.

If stress seems to trigger the symptoms, then a diary should be maintained to record the symptoms and the events associated with them. This would help clarify the connection between the two. Once the events or situations have been identified, ways to deal with them can be devised. Regular or vigorous exercise or any hobby may provide a break from stressful situations.

Diet

Eat fewer greasy, high-fat foods. Spicy foods bother some people. Instead of raw fibre, cooked fibre is better tolerated in case of an acute attack. For instance, vegetable soups are better than fruit juices; cooked vegetables are better than salads. Drink water instead of caffeine, alcohol or sugary drinks (they're intestinal stimulants). In general, the diet is based on whether the main symptom is constipation or diarrhoea.

For constipation, add fibre to your diet in the form of fresh fruits and vegetables, whole grains and pulses, and also increase the intake of water. Fibre absorbs water and softens the stools. Regular exercise also maintains bowel regularity.

For diarrhoea, limiting the intake of certain foods helps, e.g., beans, cabbage, apples, citrus fruits, milk and milk products, coffee, tea, colas, chocolate, alcohol, spicy and fried foods.

Essentially, it's getting to know about your body's tolerance or intolerance for specific foods. Keep a track of what you can tolerate. A food diary may help figure out your food intolerance. Mint in any form has been found beneficial in an acute attack.

ACIDITY

Frequent, persistent heartburn (acidity) is a big problem for many people. In this condition, the acid from the stomach splashes up into the food pipe. Medication can help control the condition, as can lifestyle changes. Stress is a common part of life's events. It is the way you react physically, mentally and emotionally to various situations. The inability to regularly release tension caused by stress may result in physical symptoms of acidity. In such cases, trying to decrease the stress and the tensions that ensue from them would result in a proportionate decrease in heartburn.

Heartburn is also one of the symptoms of indigestion. And indigestion results from eating too much or too fast, from eating when tense, tired or emotionally upset, from food that is too fatty or spicy or badly cooked.

Avoiding certain foods helps some people, who find that specific foods and drinks create problems. Others say that the amount of food and the time of the day are what matter. The proper weight needs to be maintained; overweight people should reduce their weight. Cigarettes and alcohol are best avoided.

Diet

Problem foods include fried, fatty and creamy stuff, chocolate, peppermint, garlic, onions, coffee, all colas and alcoholic beverages. These foods increase the acid content in the stomach. Foods that may irritate or damage the lining of the food pipe should be limited, e.g., citrus fruits and juices (including tomatoes and oranges), bottled/ tinned juices, chilli sauce and black pepper. Carbonated beverages cause bloating, putting pressure on the stomach and forcing the acid back into the food pipe. They should therefore be avoided.

Improving one's eating habits also reduces heartburn. After eating, an upright posture should be maintained. Meals should be moderate, taking care to avoid overeating. Dinner should be at least three hours before sleeping and bedtime snacks must be avoided. Though there are no studies to support the observation, a high-protein diet seems to result in lesser incidence of heartburn.

Chewing *saunf* (avoid *chooran*) after a meal stimulates the production of saliva, an alkaline solution that helps soothe and protect the food pipe. Even sucking a sweet stimulates the saliva, thereby reducing the time the stomach acid is in contact with the food pipe.

Tip: Eat smaller, low-fat meals and avoid the after-dinner alcoholic drink.

FLATULENCE

This is abdominal discomfort caused by the presence of air or gas, due to a high residue, spiced, vegetarian diet or an infestation of intestinal parasites. Belching or burping is the voluntary or involuntary release of air from the stomach through the mouth. Burping a couple of times after meals is normal, as swallowing some air while eating usually causes it. Everyone passes gas, some people more so than others. It is normal to pass gas ten to 15 times a day.

Apart from swallowing air while eating, the common causes of flatulence are the gas-producing foods and beverages, which should be avoided by those who are distressed by excessive gas in the abdomen.

Diet

Gas-producing foods are vegetables like onions, cabbage, cauliflower, capsicum, cucumber, radish and peas; fruits such as raw apples, apricots, bananas and melons; all kinds of beans; fried and fatty foods; sugars and sweets; milk and other dairy products for those who have trouble digesting lactose (the main sugar found in milk); carbonated drinks, beer and red wine.

The food should be chewed well, as intestinal enzymes cannot properly digest unmasticated food. Constipation should be avoided. Obese persons who eat excessive food often suffer from flatulence. Their total calorie intake should be curtailed in order to reduce flatulence and body weight.

If the flatus is foul smelling, meat products and eggs should be reduced to a minimum. Pulses are best excluded. Garlic has the property of inhibiting the growth of bacteria in the colon, thereby reducing flatulence. It should be included in the diet while cooking or taken as garlic capsules. About eight to ten glasses of fluid a day helps in regular bowel movement. Water should not be taken with meals, as it may aggravate distension. Sucking fluid through a straw or drinking directly from a bottle leads to swallowing of air and should be avoided.

Instead of taking only two meals per day, one should take three or four smaller meals. Dinner should be light and eaten at least two hours before sleeping.

CONSTIPATION

This is the most common physiological disorder of the digestive system characterised by infrequent and incomplete evacuation of hard, dried stools.

Constipation is most commonly due to:

(a) **Lack of fluids:** When perspiration is profuse and an adequate amount of fluid is not taken, the result is a small quantity of hard dry stools.

(b) **Lack of roughage:** Faulty food habits, which include irregular hours of meals, consuming inadequate fibre, fasting or avoiding vegetables, leave little residue for evacuation.

(c) **Vitamin B deficiency:** Deficient intake of vitamin B also produces loss of tone of the bowel wall.

(d) **Irregular bowel habits:** These may be due to getting up late in the morning and trying to rush through the morning rituals and breakfast, leaving very little time for a visit to the toilet before going to work.

(e) **Mental stress:** Stress and tension produce spasm of the colon, commonly seen in tense, highly-strung, apprehensive individuals.

The ritual of regularly administering purgatives to infants and children to cleanse their stomach affects the muscle tone of their intestines and ultimately leads to constipation that persists throughout life. Normal healthy children should never be given purgatives as a routine measure. Instead, extra water, juices or fruits like banana should be given.

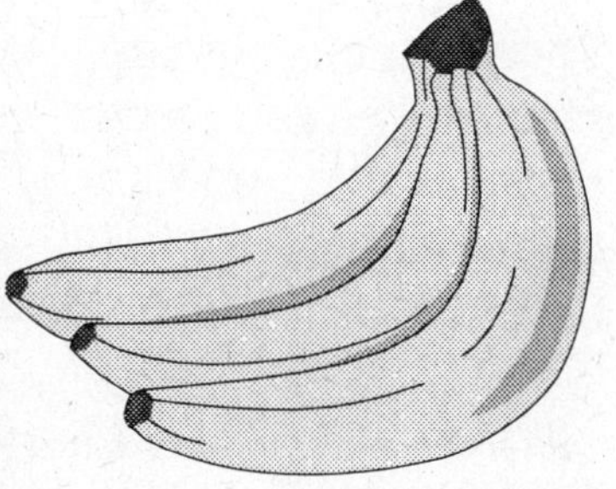

Diet

Fats stimulate the flow of bile and also lubricate the large intestine. Butter, *ghee* and cooking oils are also beneficial for lean patients. Fried foods should be avoided.

Adequate bulk (even in an obese patient on a reducing diet) can be supplied in the form of vegetables and whole fruits that are rich in unabsorbable cellulose. Unrefined cereals that contain bran can also provide bulk. In lean people, bananas, dried fruits like figs, raisins, dates and apricots are useful adjuncts.

Vitamins of the B group, preferably as yeast (*khamir*), help regulate the bowel function. Potassium in the form of vegetable soups or fruit juices also helps prevent constipation.

A liberal amount of fluids, about ten glasses or more in hot humid weather, is advised. Warm fluid taken in the early morning on an empty stomach, such as hot water or weak tea, helps some people to evacuate the bowel.

If roughage provided by green vegetables and whole fresh fruits does not relieve constipation, extra wheat bran can be added to *chapatis* to produce bulk.

There are vegetable products like *isabgol* and china grass (*agar agar*), which absorb a considerable amount of water, thereby producing a non-irritating bulk that stimulates the intestinal movement. Before retiring, about two to three teaspoons of *isabgol* can be taken with water. One tablespoon of *gulukand*, taken with a cup of warm milk, is very effective in chronic constipation.

Daily exercise, such as a game of golf or a brisk walk, is always helpful.

DIARRHOEA AND DYSENTERY

Diarrhoea means the passage of unformed stools. When unformed stools are accompanied by the passage of blood and mucous, the illness is called dysentery. The causative organism in diarrhoea and dysentery can be isolated in many patients, but in others no pathogen may be discovered in spite of a careful search. It is possible that a virus may be the cause in some instances.

Diet

Easily digestible protein-rich foods like boiled egg and skimmed milk may be given, if tolerated. In some patients, sensitive to milk and unknowingly taking large quantities, the diarrhoea comes under control only when milk and milk products are excluded from the diet.

Fats are restricted as these are not properly absorbed and may aggravate diarrhoea. Easily digestible carbohydrates such as softly cooked vegetables and soups can be given liberally.

Many patients with diarrhoea resort to self-imposed starvation, which may be harmful. In all cases of diarrhoea, whether medical facilities are available or not, it is best to start with liberal amounts of fluids like water, fresh lime juice and vegetable or *dal* soups in order to ensure an adequate intake of fluids and electrolytes.

Spices, whole pulses, fried foods and fibrous vegetables and fruits are best avoided.

Peptic Ulcers

An ulcer is defined as an open sore. Peptic ulcer is one of the most common diseases in civilised countries. An ulcer may form in any part of the digestive tract, but is mainly found in the stomach. In other words, we can say that a peptic ulcer is an open sore in the stomach. The commonest symptom of a peptic ulcer is pain or discomfort in the upper central abdomen. The pain is commonly described as burning or gnawing in character. Other symptoms that may occur are loss of weight, heartburn, acidity and vomiting.

Certain occupations appear to predispose people to ulcers. Doctors are particularly prone and so are those in responsible positions in industry, such as foremen and business executives. It has been suggested that stress and strain, and hurried and irregular meals with the consequent bolting of food and inadequate mastication might be important contributory factors. Symptoms are often relieved when a patient curtails his business and social activities. Both physical and mental rest appear to promote the healing of an ulcer.

Diet

It is usually said that a suitable diet for peptic ulcer patients should be mechanically and chemically non-irritating, and should consist of small frequent meals. However, there is little evidence to support this advice. It has been shown, for example, that hourly feeding of milk provokes more acid secretion in the stomach than does the ordinary routine of three meals a day. The reason behind this is very simple. Whenever any food is taken, be it a liquid like milk or a solid like bread, it always results in acid production by the stomach wall, which is how the digestive process functions. This implies that frequent (two hourly or six to eight in total) feeds, as suggested in the traditional ulcer regime, would result in more acid production. And if there are ulcers present, then such a feeding schedule with high acid production would certainly hamper the healing process. Thus instead of improving, the patient will become a chronic case of peptic ulcers.

There is no evidence that the rate of ulcer healing can be accelerated by the traditional bland ulcer diet. Instead, studies have shown that red chilli powder has no effect on the intensity of pain or the healing of ulcer! Persistence with frequent or bland diet or liquid diet may be harmful, since, apart from more acid production, they may also lead to sub-optimal intake of vitamin C. This vitamin is contained in all fresh fruits and vegetables, which are contra-indicated in the traditional bland ulcer regime. The reason being that these foods are mechanically irritating to the inner lining of the stomach. Many patients find that their symptoms are aggravated by certain foods or alcohol. These they learn to avoid by experience.

There are no diet restrictions for peptic ulcer patients but there is good evidence to show that stopping smoking accelerates the healing of peptic ulcers.

Ulcerative Colitis

Ulcerative colitis is a disease of unknown cause characterised by inflammation and ulceration of the large intestine (colon), resulting in the frequent passage of stools with blood and mucus. The onset resembles an attack of dysentery. The failure to respond to the usual therapeutic measures draws attention to the fact that the disease might be ulcerative colitis. This disease is more common in females.

Acute attacks are more often during mental conflicts and emotional stress. Allergy to certain foods may be a factor in precipitating the disease. Milk, for instance, is one of the foods not well tolerated by patients who suffer from this disease and its exclusion from the diet always helps.

Severe weakness in ulcerative colitis is the result of insufficient food consumption, loss of blood and electrolytes in the stools. Liver damage is not unusual in prolonged ulcerative colitis, impairing proper synthesis of proteins and storage of fat-soluble vitamins.

Diet

A soft, low-fibre, high-protein diet is recommended. This can be achieved in a person taking a mixed diet. In a vegetarian it is a difficult task, particularly when milk is also excluded.

Fat used in normal cooking is tolerated. Fried foods are not easily digested and therefore should be avoided.

All forms of irritant and stale foods should be strictly avoided. Raw salads, dried fruits and nuts, condiments and spices, *papad*, *chutney* and pickles are strictly prohibited.

Cereals should be taken in the refined form (*chokar* to be removed). Only *dhuli dals* should be consumed.

Mineral loss may be marked and unless replaced may contribute to a fatal outcome. So liberal amounts of fluid, especially in the form of soups, is advisable.

Diet in Coronary Heart Disease

Forty years ago coronary heart disease was essentially a disease of men belonging to the well-to-do classes, successful businessmen and professionals like doctors and so on. It was uncommon to find an affected woman. Since then, there has been a steady increase in the incidence of this disease affecting both the sexes of all classes.

Coronary heart disease is about ten times as common in men as in women up to the age of 45 years. After the age of 50 years, there is an increased incidence in women. By the age of 70 years, there is no difference between the sexes. Short and fat people are more susceptible. In certain cases the susceptibility is inherited. People who show an excessive sense of time urgency, a preoccupation with vocational deadlines and enhanced aggressiveness and competitive drive have increased chances of coronary heart diseases.

Over 20 studies have been done on thousands of people in 14 countries. All of them have found that the three biggest risk factors for coronary heart disease are high plasma total cholesterol, cigarette smoking and high blood pressure (hypertension). 'Cigarette smoking is injurious to health', a statutory warning on every cigarette pack means that it predisposes one to coronary heart disease. The mechanism behind it is not clear. What is clear, however, is that patients with coronary heart disease should give up smoking.

The other risk factors are diabetes, obesity and, in some cases, gout. In diet, an increased consumption of animal fats and sugar has been found to contribute to the rise of these diseases. An extraordinary finding, for which no explanation has yet been established, is that harder the drinking water, the lower is the death rate from coronary heart diseases.

Prosperity certainly leads to reduction in the amount of manual work done by a person. As the wealth of a country increases, the labour class declines and is replaced by those who flick switches and occupy office chairs. An increase in private cars and public transport reduces the number of those who rely on walking and cycling. There is certainly some evidence that physical activity protects against coronary heart diseases.

Diet

All cholesterol in blood plasma is carried on lipoproteins. Low-density lipoprotein (LDL) cholesterol, which normally carries about three-fourths of the total cholesterol, is the risk factor, as it carries cholesterol into the inner lining of the artery walls. High-density lipoprotein (HDL) cholesterol, on the contrary, tends to act as a protective factor, as it clears some of the cholesterol deposited in the periphery and carries it to the liver, where it can be excreted with the bile. Deposition of cholesterol on the inner aspect of the walls of the arteries is part of the process of formation of atherosclerosis, the pathological basis of coronary heart disease.

Plasma HDL cholesterol only makes up about one-quarter of normal total cholesterol concentration, and its level is higher in women than in men, but never very high. Total cholesterol that is high nearly always results from the elevation of LDL cholesterol. Plasma (total or LDL) cholesterol may be raised as the inherited condition of hypercholesterolemia, a condition with a tendency towards premature coronary heart disease. Plasma cholesterol is also raised secondary to certain diseases; e.g., hypothyroidism, some types of kidney disease, bile duct obstruction, and diabetes. Finally, it is moderately raised by a diet rich in saturated fat and cholesterol.

In order to lower the blood cholesterol level, the diet has to be slightly modified. Cholesterol is essentially present in all animal fats. It is not desirable to restrict all forms of fats, as severe restrictions may result in mental depression. The total intake of fat should not be more than 30 per cent of the total calorie intake. It should be consumed partly as unsaturated vegetable oils, such as mustard oil, *til* oil, groundnut oil, olive oil, etc. Saturated fats, hydrogenated vegetable oil (*vanaspati*), coconut oil, margarine and animal fats like butter, cream and *ghee* should be taken in moderation. Mutton and organ meats should be replaced by fish and chicken. The use of egg should also be restricted to two to three eggs per week. Whole milk should be replaced by skimmed milk.

Vegetables, fruits, cereals, *sabut dals*, skimmed milk and lean meat should be the main items of diet. The fibre content of the diet should be increased as much as possible. Three or four smaller meals are preferable to two big meals. The evening meal should be taken about two hours before sleeping.

In the case of high blood pressure, which is mostly associated with coronary heart diseases, a low salt diet is advised. In such a diet, no table salt is permitted, and salt used in cooking must be reduced to a minimum. All tinned and processed products containing preservatives (sauces, jams, pickles etc.) and confectionaries containing baking powder (cakes, biscuits etc.) should be avoided. The maximum number of slices of ordinary bread allowed per day is five thin slices only. Butter used should be salt free. Helpings of fresh meats, fish, potatoes and other root vegetables should be small.

Since obesity predisposes one to coronary heart diseases, it is advisable to restrict the total calorie intake to reduce weight to the expected normal for one's height, age and sex. In normal individuals, the ideal body weight should be maintained by keeping a periodic check.

Obesity is also associated with elevated total cholesterol and triglyceride levels and lower HDL levels. Even gradual increases in body fat may produce unhealthy cholesterol levels. One study found that an average increase of one kilo of fat a year, as people aged, caused total cholesterol to rise and HDL levels to drop. The goal for a cholesterol-lowering diet then must also include attaining or maintaining a healthy weight.

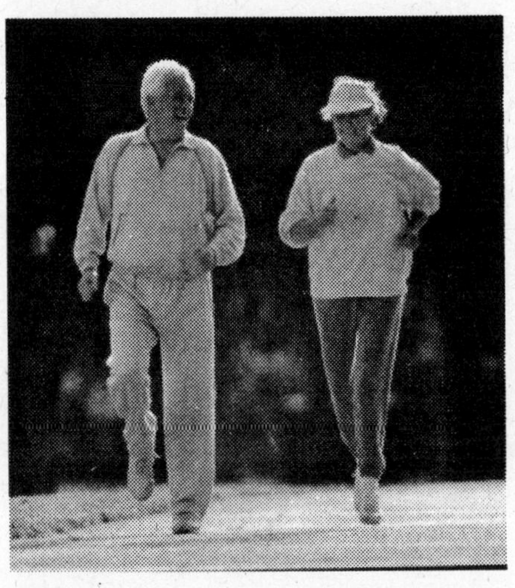

A recent study reported that dietary changes improve cholesterol levels only when an aerobic exercise programme is also included. In addition to having a beneficial effect on cholesterol, exercise is critical to maintaining a healthy heart; it helps keep weight off and lowers the heart rate and blood pressure. People who maintain an active lifestyle have a 45% lower risk of developing coronary heart disease than do sedentary people. Regular aerobic exercises — brisk walking, jogging, swimming, cycling, aerobic dance, and racquet sports — are the best forms of exercise for lowering LDL and raising HDL levels.

It may take up to a year of sustained exercise for HDL levels to show significant improvement. Experts recommend that people aim for a routine of a 30-minute brisk walk most days of the week; an excellent goal is 20 to 25 miles a week, but in terms of raising HDL levels, more is better. Resistance (weight) training offers a complementary benefit by reducing LDL levels. After a high-fat meal, triglycerides can be lowered either with a single, prolonged (about 90 minutes) aerobic session or by several shorter sessions during the day.

One study indicated, however, that short bursts of exercise actually increase LDL oxidation — the process that makes LDL dangerous to the heart, so individuals should always aim for a consistent, regular programme. Before engaging in any strenuous exercise, it is advisable to consult a physician. Children should especially be encouraged to exercise every day.

Liver Diseases

The liver is a very important organ of our body in which many metabolic processes occur. Toxins and bacteria absorbed from the intestine may directly reach the liver and cause injury. Dietary deficiencies may make the organ susceptible to the injurious effects of infections and toxins.

Methionine is an amino acid that prevents liver damage caused by any dietary deficiency. Since milk and animal proteins are rich in methionine, the consumption of milk or animal foods prevents damage of the liver cells.

Glycogen also protects the liver cells against damage. Carbohydrates are useful not only for meeting energy requirements but also for reducing the endogenous breakdown of proteins by their 'protein sparing effect'.

In general, vitamins of the B group have a beneficial effect on the liver.

Alcohol supplies calories but it cannot be stored in the liver as glycogen. When alcohol is taken there is a proportionate increase in the need for protein and vitamins of the B group. Further, the gastritis produced by alcohol may reduce the appetite and thereby the intake of proteins. A chronic alcoholic is often deficient in proteins, carbohydrates and vitamins, which makes his liver highly vulnerable to any infection or toxin.

JAUNDICE

Jaundice is the yellow discolouration of the skin with bile pigments, due to rise in the serum bilirubin. Jaundice may be produced due to excessive breakdown of red blood cells or due to the damage of the cells either by viral infection or by toxic drugs. The commonest cause of jaundice is viral hepatitis.

Viral jaundice is usually a self-limiting disease. Most patients recover with only rest, diet and vitamins. Viral hepatitis tends to run a more severe course in undernourished patients than in the well nourished.

Diet

In severe jaundice (serum bilirubin over 15 mg) a moderate intake of protein is required, through cereals like porridge, rice, biscuits, bread, rusks and *chapatis*. When the intensity of jaundice is less, or on recovery from jaundice, a high-protein diet containing *dals*, beans, eggs, fish and meat is recommended.

There is no evidence that when the usual amount of protein is taken, the average consumption of fat is harmful. In severe jaundice fat may be avoided. In moderate to mild jaundice about 50-60 gm of fat may be given daily (to be used in cooking — fried foods are not permitted).

Pickles, dried fruits and nuts should be avoided in all cases of jaundice.

Carbohydrates are necessary to provide energy and reduce the endogenous breakdown of proteins to a minimum. Fruits, fruit juice, vegetables and vegetable juices, soups, sugar, *gur*, and honey should be given liberally, as they not only provide carbohydrates but also supply adequate minerals and vitamins.

GALLSTONES

The gall-bladder is a thin-walled pouch situated on the under-surface of the liver. The liver secretes bile, which is concentrated and stored in the gall-bladder, when not required for digestion. Gallstone is the commonest disease of the gall-bladder. The incidence of gallstones is higher in women, being present in at least 20 per cent of women over the age of 40 years.

Gallstones are mainly formed of cholesterol, mixed with some bile pigments, calcium carbonate and phosphate.

Gallstones associated with attacks of severe pain or jaundice are to be treated by surgery. The mere presence of asymptomatic gallstones in the elderly, however, is not an indication for surgery. Dietetic management is necessary to prevent gallstone formation.

Diet

It is noticed that gallstones are prevalent among those communities consuming significantly more calories (gallstones being one of the many complications of obesity). The minimum number of calories to maintain normal body weight is therefore advised. Since carbohydrates contribute to excess calories, a high-carbohydrate diet should be avoided. Higher protein intake also increases biliary cholesterol concentration. A moderate protein intake is recommended. An effort should be made to maintain an ideal body weight according to the height and age.

Symptoms of bloating (gas), belching and indigestion usually ascribed to gallstones are normally due to the intolerance of fatty foods. For people in whom fats do not produce symptoms, refined vegetable oils are advised. Fried foods are to be excluded, as they would always produce discomfort.

Kidney Diseases

The kidneys excrete waste products of the body in general and the end products of protein metabolism in particular. These excretory products are retained in the body if the quantity of urine or its concentration is inadequate. Urea is one of the end products of protein metabolism, derived from ingested food and the breakdown of body tissues.

ACUTE NEPHRITIS

At the onset of acute nephritis the excretion of urine is markedly diminished. Urea and other end products of protein metabolism are retained.

Diet

A high carbohydrate, low protein, low salt diet is advised with restricted fluids. Restricting the intake of dietary proteins considerably diminishes the formation of urea and other waste products. Supplying 'protein sparers' like carbohydrates and fats reduces the breakdown of tissue proteins. The intake of proteins cannot be restricted indiscriminately, however. Adequate proteins should be supplied as soon as the kidneys recover and normal urinary flow is resumed.

Normal kidneys automatically regulate the sodium and potassium needs of the body. In acute nephritis the kidneys are unable to excrete sodium and potassium and so the body's electrolyte balance is disturbed. Mineral intake, therefore, has to be restricted. Salt is restricted as long as there is swelling (oedema). Only two helpings daily of either fruit juice or vegetable soup are permitted.

Apart from the water excreted in the urine, about one litre is also lost daily through respiration, perspiration and defecation. The daily intake of fluids and output of urine should be charted. Daily fluid replacement (including fruit juice, milk, tea and soups) should be one litre plus the daily amount excreted in the urine.

NEPHROTIC SYNDROME

This is characterised by a varying degree of proteinuria (excretion of protein in the urine) and oedema (swelling due to water retention). Serum cholesterol values are raised. The total quantity of urine excreted may be normal.

Diet

Since there is loss of protein in the urine, it leads to protein depletion of the tissues. So a high protein, moderate fat diet is advised. Salt is restricted till the oedema persists.

URINARY STONES

The kidneys, as mentioned earlier, excrete the end products of metabolism, like uric acid, phosphate and oxalate along with minerals like sodium, calcium and magnesium. If these minerals crystallise and precipitate, a stone is formed. The commonest renal stones are oxalates, urates or phosphates, combined with calcium.

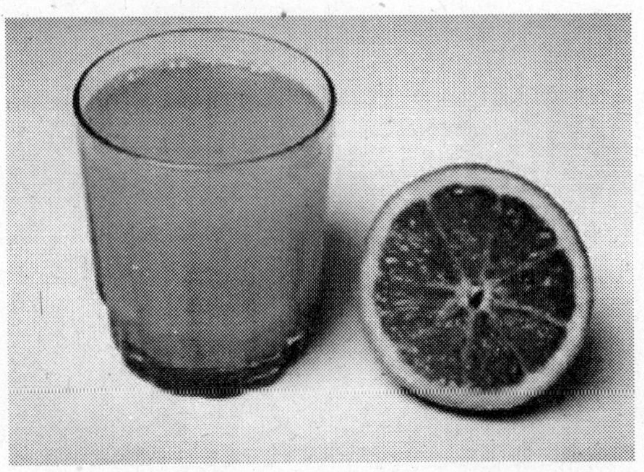

Diet

Stone formation is a gradual process extending over a long period of time and once a tendency for its formation has developed, it will persist throughout life. Vigilance with fluid intake and diet is needed indefinitely.

The fundamental principle in the treatment of urinary stones is to supply adequate fluids like water, coconut and barley water, fruit juices, thin soups and weak tea in order to ensure the passage of over two litres of urine per day. Diluted urine avoids concentration of minerals and also tends to make the urine neutral, thus preventing the strong acid or alkaline reaction that predisposes the precipitation of crystals.

Although the role of diet in the formation of urinary stones is not well established, it is advisable to restrict foods that are rich in calcium, oxalate or uric acid, according to the type of stone formed.

Foods rich in Calcium: All kinds of beans, cauliflower, potatoes, egg yolk, figs, milk and milk products (except butter and *ghee*).

Foods rich in Oxalate: Tomato, spinach, *chickoo*, custard apple, strawberries, cashewnuts, chocolates, cocoa, tea.

Foods rich in Uric Acid: Liver, kidney, salmon, sardine.

Brain-boosting Diet

How often do you forget your friends' phone numbers or where you have put the keys? Rather than blaming your dwindling memory on age, or a busy lifestyle, take a look at your diet. What you eat affects the clarity of your thoughts and level of concentration, your intelligence level, memory, and reaction time, and even how quickly your brain ages.

Though the brain makes up only two per cent of total body weight, it uses up to 30 per cent of the day's calories. Since the brain burns the fuel even while we sleep, eating breakfast is the best way to restock fuel stores and prevent mental fatigue later in the day. After two to three weeks of adding breakfast to your daily routine, you should notice a gain in energy and mental power, especially if the meal includes a fruit, a cereal (*parantha/dalia/uppama*) and a protein-rich source (milk, egg, curd, *paneer*, sprouts).

Also, spread the food intake among four to six mini-meals and snacks evenly distributed throughout the day. Keep these meals light. Avoid high-fat or big meals that divert the blood supply to the digestive tract and away from the brain, causing sluggishness and fatigue.

Crash diets do more than deprive you of calories; they make your brain sluggish. Researchers at the Institute of Food Research in the United Kingdom report that women on low-calorie diets process information more slowly, take longer to react and have more trouble remembering sequences compared with non-dieting women. In contrast, losing weight the good old-fashioned way — a gradual weight loss of no more than a kilo a week — allows you to lose fat not muscle, keep it off, and stay clear-headed in the process.

A cup of coffee helps you think and work faster and more efficiently. But too much has adverse effects. Caffeine lingers in the system for up to 15 hours. A cup of coffee or cola taken in the mid-afternoon could disrupt sleep at 10 p.m., resulting in mental fatigue and poor judgement the next day. Coffee and tea contain compounds called tannins that reduce other brain-boosting nutrients, such as iron, by up to 75%. Limit the coffee and tea intake to three cups or less each day, drinking them between meals.

Iron helps carry oxygen to the tissues, including the brain. When iron levels drop, tissues are starved of oxygen, resulting in fatigue, memory loss, poor concentration, lack of motivation, shortened attention span and reduced work performance. Menstruating women need at least 15 milligrams of iron daily, yet many consume 10 milligrams or less.

Eat more iron-rich foods, including beans and peas, dark green leafy vegetables and dried apricots. Cook in iron pots. The iron will leach out of the pot into the food, raising its iron content. Drink vitamin C-rich (lime, lemon, orange, grapefruit) juices to boost iron absorption.

Inadequate intake of any B-vitamin, including vitamins B_1, B_2, B_6, B_{12} and folic acid, literally starves the brain of energy and leads to confusion, irritability, impaired thinking, and affects concentration, memory, reaction time and mental clarity.

To boost B-vitamins, include several daily servings of vitamin B-rich foods, including toned milk and curd, bananas, whole grains, sprouts, beans and peas.

The brain consumes more oxygen than any other body tissue. This exposes the brain to a huge daily dose of free radicals, by-products of oxygen usage that attack and damage brain cells. After decades, the wear and tear of free-radical attacks can contribute to the gradual loss of memory and thinking, an effect associated with ageing. Fortunately, the body has an anti-free-radical army comprising antioxidant nutrients, which include vitamins C and E. This dietary militia deactivates the free radicals.

To keep your antioxidant defences strong, consume at least five but preferably nine servings of the following foods each day: orange juice, strawberries, carrots, spinach, and dark-coloured fresh fruits and vegetables.

Anti-stress Diet

Periods of pressure and stress, short or long, are part of everybody's life, whether caused by disturbing events (death in the family), unusual challenges (a new job) or even happy changes (promotion). You may not be aware of it but stress affects your body's ability to handle various kinds of foods.

One thing that happens when you are under stress is a sudden constriction of your blood vessels. This raises your blood pressure and also reduces the amount of blood going to your stomach and intestines. The flow of enzymes (digestive aids) is slowed as well. Much of the food you eat, particularly if it has a high fat content, is therefore poorly digested. Instead of being broken down properly, it ferments in the intestine, causing gas and distension.

Another thing that happens right away in any stress reaction is a hormonal alert that your blood needs more glucose — in other words, you feel more hungry. This may prompt you to eat a lot of carbohydrates, either sugar or starch. The reaction is an appropriate one if you are facing strenuous physical exertion, but it gives you

Physical, Emotional & Behavioural Signs of Stress		
Behavioural signs		
Do you smoke?	YES	NO
Do you have problems in sleeping?	YES	NO
Do you often get minor illnesses, like colds and flu?	YES	NO
Do you consume more alcohol than is good for you?	YES	NO
Have you had much time away from work?	YES	NO
Emotional signs		
Do you worry excessively?	YES	NO
Are you short-tempered?	YES	NO
Do you find it hard to concentrate?	YES	NO
Do you often feel anxious or fearful?	YES	NO
Are you excessively concerned about your physical health?	YES	NO
Have you lost your sense of humour?	YES	NO
Physical signs		
Do you notice your heart racing?	YES	NO
Do you often get headaches?	YES	NO
Do you sometimes feel breathless or faint?	YES	NO
Do you sometimes feel hot and sweaty?	YES	NO
Do you often get indigestion or diarrhoea?	YES	NO
Do you often get a dry mouth?	YES	NO

Note : *The more questions you answered 'yes', the more likely you are to have a stress problem — although you may have been unaware of it.*

only surplus calories (increase in weight) if the stress is psychological.

Here are some helpful pointers you can follow for an anti-stress diet:

- Cut down on table salt and other sources of sodium because of their link with high blood pressure. Remember that preservatives may also contain sodium.
- Drink only moderate amounts of coffee and tea and remember that caffeine is present in both. Caffeine, nicotine and alcohol are stimulants.
- You should have eight big glasses of fluids in a day. It can be in the form of any drink, but make sure you drink at least two glasses of plain water daily. This helps to flush waste products out of the body.
- Eat foods that are rich in potassium, like oranges and bananas. Potassium is essential for the right balance of the minerals within body fluids and plays a key role in muscle contraction.
- Be sure you are getting enough calcium, as you tend to lose more than usual when you are in a stressful situation. You should try to have at least two glasses of skimmed/toned (reduced fat content) milk in a day.
- Vitamin C is important, as it keeps the walls of the capillaries flexible. The blood vessels constrict at the first sign of stress, and this results in the depletion of vitamin C in the body. Sources of vitamin C are the citrus fruits (orange, lime, lemon, grapefruit) and fresh vegetables eaten raw as salad.

- The vitamin B complex serves as a catalyst in the production of energy, and in the metabolism of protein and fats. It is also necessary for the working of the central nervous system. In conditions of stress (especially physical), supplements are advisable. Increase the intake of green leafy vegetables, eggs, milk, whole grains, sprouts and yeast (*khameer*).

- Nitrogen, the base of the body's protein, is excreted under stress. So the protein intake should be increased by 10% during a stress period.

- Five small meals are lighter than three large ones on the digestive system. The additional small meals can take the form of afternoon or evening snacks.

- Relax before a meal. Sit down at the table for every meal, putting your worries aside.

- Try and include apples (with the skin), apricots, bananas, French beans, cabbage, cauliflower, cherries, corn, grapefruit, lemon, lettuce, melons, mushrooms, ladies' fingers, oranges, peaches, pears, peas, pineapple, plums, potatoes, rice and tomatoes in your diet. They are high potassium and low sodium foods.

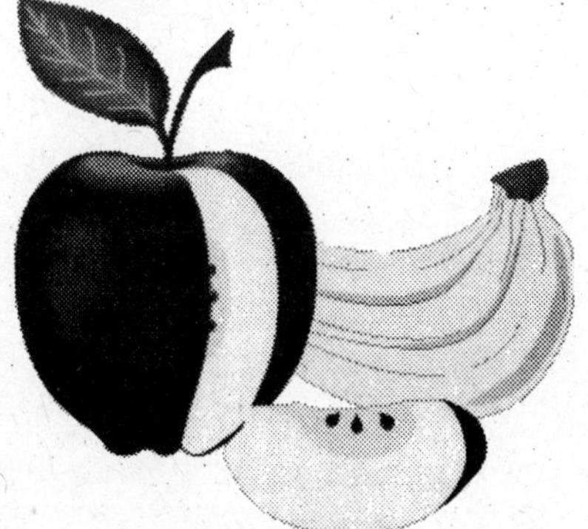

Relief in Hot Flashes

Not all women want to take hormone replacement therapy, although it's known to make menopausal life better — especially the hot flashes. Instead, the diet can be modified to eradicate the flashes.

Soybean has been found to give hot-flash relief. Eating or drinking two servings of soy a day – in the forms of soybean *dal*, nuggets, soymilk or tofu, takes 4 to 6 weeks to show the effect.

Avoiding certain foods can also give relief in hot flashes. Hot and spicy foods and hot drinks (tea, coffee) should be avoided. Also, avoid large meals as they increase the body temperature, especially meals that are high in fat.

Healthy Recipes

SOUPS

Mixed Vegetable Soup

Serves 4

1 medium-sized carrot, diced

1 medium-sized onion, diced

2 medium-sized potatoes, diced

¼ small cabbage, finely shredded

2 cloves garlic, crushed

Salt and pepper to taste

750 ml water

150 ml skimmed milk

1 tbsp chopped coriander

Simmer the vegetables, except the cabbage, in water for half an hour, or until the vegetables are tender. Add the cabbage and continue cooking for ten minutes. Add the milk, reheat and add the coriander. Adjust seasoning if necessary and serve.

Red Bean Soup

Serves 4

30 ml corn oil

2 medium-sized onions, chopped

2 medium-sized carrots, diced

Any other seasonal vegetable(s), diced

100 gm *rajma* beans, soaked

200 gm tomatoes

2 litres water

A small piece of cinnamon and a bay leaf

Salt to taste

Heat the oil in a large pan; add the beans and all the vegetables, except the tomatoes. Cover and cook gently for about 15 minutes. Add the tomatoes, water, salt, cinnamon and bay leaf; bring to boil, then simmer for approximately an hour.

For variety, other beans can be substituted for *rajma* beans.

Italian Vegetable Soup

Serves 4

100 gm beans (any), soaked

1 medium-sized onion, chopped

2 cloves garlic, crushed

2 young spring onions, chopped

2 medium-sized carrots, sliced

200 gm snake-gourd (*tori*), sliced

200 gm tomatoes

200 gm potatoes, chopped with skin on
¼ small cabbage, finely shredded
100 gm fresh peas
100 gm pasta (any)
3-4 leaves of fresh basil (*tulsi*)
A pinch of mixed herbs/oregano
Salt to taste
30 gm processed cheese, grated

Simmer the beans for 20 to 30 minutes in 2 litres of water. Add the onions, garlic, carrots, peas and potatoes, and simmer for a further half-hour. Add the cabbage, *tori*, tomatoes, pasta, salt and seasoning and continue simmering for 20 minutes or until the pasta is tender. Just before serving, sprinkle the cheese on the top.

SALADS

Bean and Cucumber Salad

Serves 4

15 ml refined oil
2 medium-sized onions, chopped
1 clove garlic, crushed
15 ml brown vinegar
30 ml lemon juice
250 gm cucumbers, diced
3 medium-sized tomatoes, chopped
Salt, pepper, mustard powder to taste
250 gm boiled *moong* beans or sprouts
2 tbsp chopped fresh coriander

Heat the oil in a pan and cook the onion and garlic gently for ten minutes. Add the vinegar and lemon juice and simmer for five minutes. Add the cucumber, tomatoes and seasoning; and stir in the beans, cool, transfer to a shallow serving dish, sprinkle with coriander and serve.

Potato Salad

Serves 4

250 gm potatoes, boiled and diced

50 gm chopped capsicum

100 gm boiled peas

75 gm curd, beaten

1 clove garlic, ground with salt

2 tbsp chopped spring onions, including green parts or chopped mint

Mix together the salad ingredients. Add the garlic to the curd and mix with the salad. Serve the salad sprinkled with chopped spring onions/mint.

Tossed Salad in Orange and Lemon Dressing

Serves 4

1 medium-sized apple, peeled, cored and diced

1 banana, sliced

Slices of 1 orange, with the skin and seeds removed

100 gm seedless grapes

100 gm pineapple, diced

100 gm cucumber, diced

1 medium-sized capsicum, diced

100 gm *paneer*, diced (optional)

Dressing:

15 ml olive oil

10 ml brown vinegar

30 ml orange juice

5 ml lemon juice

Salt and pepper to taste

Mix all the ingredients together. Beat the salad dressing ingredients together and add to salad tossing well. Leave for 15 to 20 minutes in the fridge before serving.

MAIN DISHES

Mushroom Kebabs

Serves 4

450 gm button mushrooms

150 gm curd

1 tbsp refined oil

1 tbsp lemon juice

1 tsp lemon rind

1 tsp crushed bay leaf

1 tbsp thyme

1 clove garlic, crushed

Seasoning (salt, chillies, etc.) to taste

Trim stalks from mushrooms. Put the curd in a large bowl, beat in the oil, lemon rind and juice and stir in the bay leaf, thyme, garlic and seasoning. Add the mushrooms and leave to marinate at room temperature for two hours, turning several times. Thread mushrooms on to kebab skewers and place under a hot grill for four minutes or until cooked. Serve with the remaining marinade as a dip.

Vegetables Stuffed Potatoes

Serves 4

½ kg potatoes, boiled

50 gm processed cheese, grated

1 large carrot, grated

1 large onion, chopped

1 small green pepper, chopped

Salt, black pepper powder, mustard powder to taste

Tomato rings to garnish

Onion rings to garnish

A few sprigs of coriander to garnish

Heat the oven to 200-degree C

Slice the potatoes carefully from the top, and scoop them out to make into *katoris*. Mash the scooped-out potatoes and add the vegetables and seasoning to it. Add half of the grated cheese into this mixture. Fill up the potato scoops with the mixture. Top the filled potatoes with the remaining grated cheese. Bake till the cheese starts turning golden. Serve garnished with onion and tomato rings, and sprigs of fresh coriander.

Pasta Italiana

Serves 4

200 gm macaroni
2 tbsp refined oil
2 medium-sized onions, chopped
2 cloves garlic, crushed
1 tbsp oregano
Salt and pepper to taste
2 medium-sized tomatoes, chopped
2 small carrots, sliced, boiled
100 gm beans, chopped, boiled
100 gm peas, shelled, boiled
25 gm processed cheese, grated
Heat the oven to 180-degree C

Boil the macaroni in salted water for 10 minutes and drain. Wash with cold water and keep it aside. Meanwhile, heat the oil and cook the onion and garlic slowly until tender and golden. Stir in the oregano, tomatoes, carrots, beans, peas and seasoning and cook for five minutes. Combine the pasta and vegetables, put in a baking dish, sprinkle the grated cheese on the top, and cook till the cheese turns golden brown.

Chilli Con Carne

Serves 4

2 tbsp refined oil
2 medium-sized onions, chopped
1 clove garlic, crushed

150 gm lean minced meat
2 tbsp wholemeal flour
2 tbsp tomato puree
Chilli powder to taste
1 tsp Tabasco sauce (optional)
250 gm tomatoes, chopped
250 gm *rajma* beans, soaked, boiled
Cinnamon, a small stick
2 pieces black cardamom
Salt to taste
1 medium green pepper, chopped

Heat the oil and gently fry onions and garlic for five minutes. Add the flour and salt to the meat. Add this mixture to the onions and cook until brown, stirring constantly. Mix tomato puree with chilli powder, and Tabasco sauce. Add to the meat, when it is cooked. Add chopped tomatoes, cinnamon and cardamom to beans and boil for five minutes. Mix the meat and beans, add the chopped green pepper to the mixture, cover tightly and simmer gently for 10 to 15 minutes. Ten minutes before serving stir in salt and the green pepper.

Note: *You may use soy granules instead of minced meat.*

Mixed Beans and Vegetable Casserole

Serves 4

200 gm mixed beans (*rajma*, *moong*, *urad*, *lobia*, etc.) soaked, boiled
1 tbsp refined oil

1 large onion, finely chopped

1 clove garlic, crushed

2 medium-sized green peppers, diced

2 medium-sized carrots, diced

Salt and seasoning to taste

4 medium-sized tomatoes, halved

Heat the oil and gently cook the onion and garlic until golden brown. Stir in all the vegetables and beans and cook over a low heat for 10 minutes. Add the tomatoes, salt and seasoning and cook gently for 10 minutes. Serve on a bed of boiled rice.

Lentil and Cheese Pie

Serves 4

200 gm brown lentils (*sabut masoor*), boiled

100 gm dry peas, boiled

2 tbsp refined oil

2 medium-sized onions, chopped

2 medium-sized carrots, grated

1 small green pepper, chopped

1 clove garlic, crushed

1 small piece ginger, grated

Salt and seasoning to taste

4 medium-sized tomatoes, sliced

Topping:

1 tbsp chopped onion retained from above

250 gm mashed potatoes

50 gm cheese (processed or cottage), grated

4 tbsp milk

Grated nutmeg, a pinch

Heat the oven to 200-degree C

Heat the oil and cook the onion, garlic and ginger gently for five minutes (retain 1 tbsp for the topping). Stir in the rest of the vegetables and seasoning, lower the heat and cook slowly for ten minutes.

Mix the boiled lentils and peas and mash lightly. Stir in the vegetables. Put the mixture into a large pie dish and cover with sliced tomatoes.

To make the topping, add the sautéed onion, 3 tbsp milk (retaining a little to brush on the top), cheese and seasonings to the mashed potato and mix well. Spread over the tomatoes and brush over with the remaining milk. Bake for about 30 minutes.

DESSERTS

Nutty Loaf

Makes 12 slices

150 gm plain flour

Pinch of salt

¼ tsp mixed spice

1 tsp cinnamon, powdered

75 gm polyunsaturated margarine

2 tsp grated orange rind

1 egg, beaten

90 ml skimmed milk

100 gm mixed nuts, chopped

Heat the oven to 160-degree C

Mix the flour, salt and spices. Cream the margarine and orange rind together. Fold in the flour. Add the egg and milk to the flour mixture a little at a time and beat well. Fold in the nuts. Bake for 20 to 25 minutes. Turn onto a wire rack to cool. Serve as slices.

Pears in Lime Jelly

Serves 4

20 gm unflavoured gelatine

600 ml lime squash

250 gm pears, chopped

Dissolve the gelatine in a little hot (but not boiling) water in a cup. Add the squash. When the liquid is cold, add the chopped pears. Pour into a mould or individual moulds or glass dishes and leave to set.

Strawberry Tarts

Makes 20

Pastry:

200 gm plain flour

100 gm polyunsaturated margarine

Pinch of salt

Filling:

200 gm small strawberries

200 gm skimmed milk cheese

200 ml strawberry jelly

Heat the oven to 200-degree C

Rub the margarine into the flour and salt mixture till it resembles fine breadcrumbs. Add water, little at a time, and knead it into dough. Divide and cut into 20 rounds with a fluted cutter. Press into small patty tins and bake for 10 to 15 minutes. Leave to cool, then divide the cheese between them and arrange the strawberries on top. Spoon 1 tbsp of jelly, which should be cold and just beginning to set, over the strawberries on each tartlet before serving.

Apple Crumble

Serves 4 to 6

500 gm cooking apples, cored

¼ to ½ tsp ground cloves

Sugar-free liquid sweetener to taste

4 tbsp hot water

4 tbsp rolled oats

100 gm wholemeal flour

30 gm polyunsaturated margarine

Heat the oven to 180-degree C

Slice the apples in crosscut pieces to avoid long strips of peel. Place in a baking dish, sprinkle with the cloves, and add the sweetener to taste. Mix the oats and flour together and rub in the margarine. Sprinkle over the fruit and bake for 30 to 40 minutes.

Note: *Plums can be used in place of apples. Crushed nuts can be added to give a crunchier flavour.*

Helpful Hints

Though precise rules of nutrition were not formulated in ancient days, our ancestors had evolved a set of healthy food habits such as the use of unrefined cereals, the combination of cereals and *dals* to provide 'complete' proteins, and the use of natural sugars. Modern man, however, has acquired artificial tastes and alienated himself from Nature even in his food habits. The growing consumption of refined grains, white sugar and 'junk food' creates disorders in the human body.

- Soaking, sprouting and fermentation increase the nutritional value of *dals* and cereal grains. Sprouting breaks down proteins and starches into simple forms and makes the vitamins available for ready absorption. The increase in vitamins B and C compensates for the minor losses in roasting and cooking. *Methi* seeds are especially benefited by this method. Sprouting makes them lose their bitterness, thus allowing us to avail their valuable amino acids.
- Another golden rule is combination. Since the Indian diet relies heavily on cereals, combine cereals with *dals* for maximum

protein value. Good sources of vegetable proteins are yeast (*khameer*), skimmed milk powder, soya granules, mushrooms, sprouted *dals*, peanuts and *paneer*.

- Do not over-wash vegetables, do not soak them in water for a long time, and do not store them for longer than necessary. This helps vegetables retain valuable water-soluble vitamins and minerals.

- Conserve vitamins by cooking vegetables in very little water, with a lid on the saucepan.

- Never throw away the water in which vegetables were cooked. Use it for making *dals*, curries, soups and gravies.

- Use non-stick pans to minimise the use of oil.

- Avoid using aluminium saucepans, unless you are careful not to scour them. Try to use stainless steel or enamel saucepans for soups, etc. Copper and brass vessels are highly recommended.

- As far as possible, do not liquidise vegetables and fruits at high speeds. Even *chutneys* are best ground on a grindstone, because high-speed mixers can destroy vitamins B and C.

- Do not peel fruits and vegetables unnecessarily (except for fruits such as oranges, mangoes and bananas). Peeling removes much of the nutrients that fruits and vegetables are supposed to provide.

Vitamins vs Diseases
(Diseases for which Vitamins are Recommended)

Disease	Vitamin	Disease	Vitamin
Arthritis	: 'C'	Hair	: 'B-1'
Anaemia	: 'B-6' and 'D'	Heart	: 'E'
Appetite	: 'B-1'	Infection	: 'C'
Arteries (Hardening)	: 'B-6'	Irritability, Insomnia	: 'B-6'
Beri-Beri	: 'B-1'	Kidney Stone	: 'A'
Bleeding	: 'C'	Limbs (Bleeding)	: 'C'
Blindness	: 'A' & 'D'	Menses	: 'E'
Blood Clotting, Liver Problems	: 'K'	Muscles (Pain)	: 'E' and 'B-1'
Blood Pressure	: 'E'	Myopia	: 'D'
Cataract	: 'C'	Nails	: 'B-1'
Calcium Deficiency	: 'D'	Nervous Tension	: 'B-1'
Children (for strength)	: 'A'	Pain (Body)	: 'E'
Cramp	: 'B-Complex'	Pernicious Anaemia	: 'B-12'
Constipation	: 'B-1'	Reproduction	: 'A' and 'E'
Colds	: C	Retina (Detachment)	: 'A' and 'E' (a combination of both)
Diarrhoea	: 'B-6'	Resistance	: 'A', 'B-6' & 'C'
Dry Skin, Eczema	: 'A' & 'C'	Rickets	: 'C'
Emotional Disturbance	: 'B-6'	Skin	: 'B-1' & 'B-2'
Eyes	: 'A', 'B-2' & 'E'	Stone (Kidney)	: 'A'
Fatigue	: 'B-1'	Tiredness	: 'B-12'
Gall-Bladder Stone	: 'B-6'	Thyroid Gland	: 'B-1'
Genitals	: 'A' and 'E'	Weakness	: 'D' and 'B-6'
Gums (Bleeding)	: 'C'	Weak Bones	: 'D'

A BALANCED DIET

We have all seen by now the danger of being overweight. Obesity causes high blood pressure, heart disease and many other problems, which can, in the long run, prove fatal. Being underweight on the other hand is another health hazard, causing fatigue, predisposition to disease and infection, hair and skin problems. How do you strike a balance?

Regardless of our body weight, we need to eat certain foods in specific proportions every day. According to the nutrients they contribute, the various foods can be divided into seven groups.

- The first group consists of milk and its products. An adult requires 2 to 3 servings of milk or its products everyday, and a child needs to have a minimum of 4 servings of milk daily. Besides providing good quality protein, milk also gives us calcium (for the bones and teeth) and vitamin B complex.

- The second group contains fats and oils (including butter, cream, vanaspati, *ghee*, etc.). The minimum daily fat/oil intake should be 3 tablespoons. This is chiefly the energy-providing group.

- The third group is that of cereals. These are valuable for protein, iron, B complex vitamins and calories. They provide roughage that allows easy bowel movement and keeps the digestive system in order. Items include various types of bread, *chapatis*, *idli*, *dosa*, macaroni, noodles, rice etc. Any of these should be taken in every major meal, i.e., 3 servings per day.

- The fourth group is that of proteins (body building) and contains meat, fish and poultry for non-vegetarians and nuts, *dals* and beans for vegetarians. One serving from this group is a must in our daily diet.

- The fifth group is a provider of vitamin A (for eyes) and iron (blood formation). This includes all the green leafy vegetables like spinach, mint etc. Besides maintaining the health of eyes and the skin, these vegetables have roughage enough for regular elimination (bowel) habits. One or more servings of this group are essential in our daily diet.

- The sixth group contains all the remaining vegetables and fruits. One or more servings of this group is also essential in our diet everyday. This group is a provider of all the vitamins and minerals that are essential for the normal functioning of our body system, which in turn is responsible for the healthy glow on our face, shine in our eyes and the health of our hair.

- The last group is an important group, since it provides us with vitamin C. This vitamin is necessary for the health of our gums and blood vessels. It also protects us from contracting any kind of infections, especially cold and cough. Vitamin C sources are all citrus fruits like oranges and lemons, tomatoes, amla and guava. Even green chillies and capsicum are rich in vitamin C. A daily serving of this group is desired.

Out of the above, there is no group which provides all the essentials, that is why a serving of every group is necessary in our daily diet to maintain a balance among all the nutrients.

So keeping the various food groups in mind, it becomes very simple to have a balanced diet. Sugar is not mentioned in the seven groups since it provides only empty calories and does not come under the category of essential food items.

■ ■ ■

Foods for Long Life and Well-Being

The right nutrients can add zest and health to our golden years. But the time to start eating them is now. If you've made it this far in life, chances are strong that you may live into your 80s or even 90s. But will you be living *well*? So what's the secret of staying healthy as you get older? Exercise, of course. Also, the right food. To get started, add these five nutrients to your diet.

Soy to manage cholesterol

Adding soy to your diet does not mean using more soy sauce. It means adding soy foods such as soybean flour added to the normal wheat flour, nutri nuggets, tofu, soy milk, etc. Adding soy to the diet has been shown to significantly lower the cholesterol, which reduces the risk of heart disease. Plus, soy is high in iron, which women need. Some women also say that soy helps them manage hot flashes and other symptoms of menopause. Indeed, the right diet can lower cholesterol as much as medication, according to a study reported in July 2003 in

The Journal of the American Medical Association. This four-week study found that a diet of soy fibre, protein from oats and barley, almonds, and margarine from plant sterols lowered cholesterol as much as *statins,* the most widely prescribed cholesterol medication. Soybeans actually provide high-quality protein, are low in saturated fat and contain no cholesterol, making them an ideal heart-healthy food. To lower your cholesterol, it is suggested you eat 30-40gms of soy protein everyday.

Fibre for the whole body

Once upon a time, our diet was mostly made up of whole foods that were loaded with fibre, which helped keep our cholesterol and blood sugar levels low, and kept our bowels functioning smoothly. Now in our frenzied lifestyle, we're more likely to grab fast foods or use easy-to-prepare foods at home that have negligible dietary fibre. We eat barely half the recommended amount of fibre. Studies have shown that dietary fibre — including foods such as apples, barley, beans, and other legumes, fruits and vegetables, oatmeal, oat bran, and brown rice — definitely lower the blood cholesterol. High-fibre foods are also digested slowly. So they don't cause spikes in blood sugar levels like white bread, potatoes and sweets. Also high-fibre foods help us feel full, making it easier to control weight.

Antioxidant 'Superfoods' as protectors

Superfoods are foods that are usually deep blue, purple, red, green, or orange in colour. The carotenoids and anthocyanins that provide the colour to these foods contain health-enhancing nutrients (antioxidants) that protect against heart disease and cancer and also improve our sense of balance, memory and other cognitive skills.

- **Deep green** — Cruciferous vegetables like broccoli help prevent colon cancer, while spinach is a good source of calcium.
- **Red** — Red tomatoes, especially when cooked, are beneficial sources of lycopeine, which helps protect against prostate and cervical cancer.
- **Orange/yellow** — Pumpkin, carrots, sweet potatoes, and yams promote healthy lungs and help to fightskin cancers such as *Squamous cell carcinoma.*
- **Deep blue/purple** — Brinjal, plums, blueberries, blackberries, strawberries, raspberries, and cherries lower the risk of heart disease by helping the liver clean-up extra cholesterol, as well as improve mental functioning.

Calcium for bones

As you get older, the amount of minerals in your bones decreases. Too little calcium increases your risk for *Osteoporosis* and, with it, disabling or life-threatening fractures.

If you want to keep your bones strong and lessen your chance of fractures as you get older, add calcium-rich foods such as low-fat cheese and milk to your diet. Calcium also keeps your teeth strong, helps muscles contract and helps the heart beat function properly. Recent studies have shown that calcium may even lower your risk of *Colon polyps* and help you lose weight. Dairy products are the best source of calcium. Choose skim milk, low-fat yoghurt, and low-fat cheese to avoid saturated fats. A single serving can provide you with 20% of the 1,200 milligrams a day, you need. Foods such as whole grains, dried beans and sesame seeds (til) also contain calcium. While you're adding calcium to your diet, don't forget to exercise. Take the stairs, park at the far end of the parking lot, walk wherever you can. That helps the calcium to do its job. Calcium supplements also help but since calcium-rich foods are also good sources of protein, they work much better in giving strength to the muscles supporting the bones.

Water for flushing out toxins

Water is needed to flush out toxins, keep the tissues hydrated, maintain skin tone and keep our energy up. Water is also essential if you're eating high-fibre foods, as it helps the fibre to do its job. Fibre needs water to swell up and absorb the toxins like a sponge. Don't skip water just because you don't want to get up in the middle of the night to use the bathroom, just be strategic about when you drink it. Drinking throughout the day, and not just before you go to bed should keep you from getting up during the night. If plain water doesn't quite appeal to you, add slices of lemon, lime, or orange for flavour without calories or try any mild herbal/green tea.

■ ■ ■

Improve Your Health at Work

Eight to nine hours on a chair in front of a computer, six days a week can take a toll on your body.

Tips that will help you stay healthy and in shape at work:

1. The snacks that you and your co-workers may indulge in are likely to add a few hundred calories to your daily diet if you're not careful and can leave you with unwanted kilos. The most common office-time snacks are *samosas*, *pakoras*, burgers and French fries. Try eating fruits, vegetable sandwiches, *dhoklas* or steamed momos, instead of fried foods. Have *nimbu paani* instead of soft aerated drinks.

2. Drinking adequate amount of water, i.e., eight to ten glasses everyday can help keep you hydrated. The 3 o'clock lull that many people feel at work is due to dehydration. Many foods are also good sources of water; fruits like oranges, grapes and apples can help you to remain healthy and hydrated.

3. One of the most important things, you can do during the day to stay healthy and in shape is to exercise. Walking during lunch burns calories and also helps in de-stressing. Find a walking partner whom you can depend on for a daily walk i.e., someone, who will drag you out even if you claim you're too busy. Other than walking, make it a habit to take the stairs instead of the elevator.

4. Eating a healthy lunch is an important part of a balanced diet. But eating reasonable portions is also an important part of your health. Be careful that you aren't consuming too much and then sitting on the chair, the whole day.

5. *Tension Neck Syndrome* (TNS) can occur when the neck and upper shoulders are held in a fixed, awkward position for long periods of time. It can happen to people, who talk on phone for most of the day or type a lot. *Tension Neck Syndrome* can cause neck and shoulder pain, muscle tightness and tenderness. So use a speakerphone, a shoulder cradle or use a headset at work when you're on the phone.

6. Eyestrain is another problem that is encountered in front of a computer. It can cause headaches, difficulty in focusing and increased sensitivity to light. To prevent eyestrain, the distance to the screen from your eyes should be about an arms length away. You should be able to comfortably read what's on your screen at that distance,

without having to squint. If you can't read your screen from an arm's length away, simply increase the font size on your computer.

7. Vacations are an important part of staying healthy at work. It helps you to recharge your 'batteries,' help reduce stress and get your mind off work, especially if you're having a conflict, such as problems with your boss, a co-worker or a project. Stress can impair your immune system, increasing the risk of illness, so minimizing it is essential — and vacations are just the way to do that.

8. Another way to stay healthy at work is to avoid long stretches of work in one day. Occasionally, people focus on the task at hand for too long in getting a project done and they aren't aware of the impact it's having on their health. They may not be aware of it until the stress is at a really high level, and it's affecting their relationships and their moods. This is another type of stress, commonly referred to as 'burnout'. *Burnout* can also impair a person's immune system, as well as interfere with sleep and his or her ability to concentrate.

9. Your keyboard, mouse, and phone can harbour thousands of germs that are just waiting to make you sick. According to the *Science Daily*, researchers at the 100th General Meeting of the American Society for Microbiology reported, "We know that

viruses can survive (remain infectious) for hours to days on a hard surface ... if a virus such as the *Rotavirus* (a diarrhoeal virus) were on the surface of a telephone receiver, infectious doses could easily be transferred to persons using the telephone." So get out the disinfectant and clean the machines that you use every month or rather, everyday.

10. The most important way to stay healthy at work starts with self-awareness. Know yourself and know your limits and do the best you can to stay within those limits in your job. Know when to take breaks and know when to take a vacation. And get plenty of exercise, which would help you both physically and mentally, both at work and at home.

■■■

Organic Eating

For the last many years, we have been hearing about the benefits of *vegetarianism*. 'Going green' was the thing to do. Now it is the *organic wave* that has hit us. So now when we are trying to eat healthy, choosing plenty of fresh fruits, vegetables and whole grains, we realize that there's another choice to make: Should we buy organic?

Experts say organic food is safer, more nutritious and often better tasting than non-organic food. They also say organic production is better for the environment and kinder to animals. Our very own *Ayurveda* has always prescribed organic food.

What is Organic?

Organic crops are produced without conventional pesticides or herbicides, synthetic fertilizers, sewage sludge, bioengineering or ionizing radiation. Organically raised animals are given organic feed and kept free of growth hormones and antibiotics. Organic farm animals have access to the outdoors for grazing, too.

Is Organic food safer?

In the case of pesticides, the evidence is pretty conclusive. In a large-scale study done by the **Department of Soil Science at Washington State University,** researchers looked at data from more than 94,000 food samples and 20 different crops. They found that organically grown crops consistently had about one-third as many pesticide residues as the conventionally grown versions. Organic foods also were far less likely to contain residues of more than one pesticide.

Pesticides aren't the only threats to food safety. There is also the question of natural toxins produced by the plants themselves. Because organic production steers clear of synthetic insecticides and herbicides, organic crops usually contend with more pests and weeds than conventional crops. This means that organic plants may have to produce more natural toxins. These natural pesticides could be just as harmful to people — or even more so — than the synthetic pesticides used in conventional agriculture. One familiar example is *solanine*, a substance produced by potatoes as they turn green, which can make us ill if we ingest too much of it.

Another safety concern that has been raised about organic food is the use of manure. Some critics fear that using manure to fertilize organic crops might increase the risk of contamination by dangerous microbes like *E. coli*. But organic production standards do include strict rules on the composition and application of manure. And there is not much evidence that organic food has bacterial contamination, as it generally happens because of improper handling after the food has left the farm, and conventional food is just as likely to be affected.

Whether the issue is bacterial contamination or pesticide residues, the best way to safeguard ourselves is to thoroughly rinse *all* fruits and vegetables under running water. Items with inedible skins, like melons and citrus fruits, should also be washed thoroughly because cutting the rind with a knife can bring the contaminants inside the fruit.

Is Organic food more nutritious?

A few studies have reported that organic produce has higher levels of vitamin C, certain minerals and antioxidants — thought to protect the body against ageing, cardiovascular diseases and cancer. But nutrients like vitamin C get oxidized or destroyed over time. So even though the nutrients might be higher in organic foods to begin with, if we do not eat them fresh, we lose that benefit.

Is it worth the trouble?

Whether or not organic food really is safer or more nutritious, there is one compelling reason to go organic: the health of the environment and society as a whole.

Toxic and persistent pesticides do accumulate. They accumulate in the soil; they accumulate in the water and they accumulate in our bodies. So, by eliminating the use of these pesticides and fertilizers in the organic production system, we are contributing in reducing the pollution.

But food experts caution that while the big picture is important, you must make the decision that makes the most sense for *you*. If you can manage the higher price, and you like the idea of fewer pesticides and a more environmentally friendly production system, organic food may be for you. But don't skimp on healthy conventional foods just because you think you need to save for the few organic items that you can afford.

One of the main concerns is that organic foods are more expensive. Perhaps, this is true in some instances because organic products must adhere to stricter regulations for growing, harvesting, transporting and storage; they are managed on a smaller scale and are labour intensive. However, if you weigh the costs associated with the clean-up of the country's water supply, replacement of eroded soil and health care of farmers exposed to harmful chemicals, organic foods would probably cost the same or possibly less.

■ ■ ■